Healing with
Color Zone
Therapy

by
Joseph Corvo &
Lilian Verner-Bonds

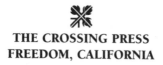

THE CROSSING PRESS
FREEDOM, CALIFORNIA

For information on bulk purchases or group discounts for this
and other Crossing Press titles, please contact our Special Sales
Manager at 800/777-1048.

Visit our Web site on the Internet: www.crossingpress.com

***In conjunction with following the recommendations in this book,
you should always follow the instructions of your doctor when
dealing with any serious health condition.***

Library of Congress Cataloging-in-Publication Data

Corvo, Joseph.
    Healing with color zone therapy / by Joseph Corvo & Lilian Verner-
Bonds.
        p. cm.
    Includes index.
    ISBN 0-89594-925-3 (pbk.)
    1. Color--Therapeutic use. I. Verner-Bonds, Lilian. II. Title.
RZ414.6.C67   1998
615.8'31--dc21   98-12119
                                                  CIP

CONTENTS

TWO MEN LOOKED
THROUGH PRISON BARS
ONE SAW MUD
THE OTHER SAW STARS

This book is dedicated to all those who seek to
understand the definition of negativity and positivity

Preface

WELCOME to the exciting world of Color Zone Therapy. Color Zone Therapy is a unique and simple system of treatment that can eliminate illness, pain and tiredness; help you to look and feel younger; and enable you to meet life with energy, vigour and vitality. In other words, it can help you to enter a new phase in your life: to become well and to stay well.

BE YOUR OWN HEALER

With the Color Zone method you can be your own healer. Everyone can use this system, and it only requires a modest input of time and effort. You can comprehensively combat pain and illness, and create lasting wellbeing. This treatment can be self-administered or given to someone else with complete confidence, and without any special training other than reading this book and following its instructions. By your own efforts, you will be eliminating not only disease, but also the cause of disease. And the methods in this book are totally complementary to any conventional forms of medical treatment that you may be receiving at present, or which you may have received in the past, so there will be no conflict between this treatment and your doctor's advice. Indeed, it is important to continue any conventional medical treatment that you are undergoing; Color Zone Therapy will form an adjunct to this.

WHAT THIS BOOK CONTAINS

In this book we will introduce ourselves and our work together. We will describe the basics of the two therapies, and show how they combine to offer a form of therapy that treats the whole person—the physical, the emotional and the spiritual body. We show you how to put it into practice with an A–Z section covering ailments commonly encountered today. Each ailment has full instructions and a chart, to enable you to treat yourself successfully. Also included in the book is a simple ten-minute-a-day routine for overall health maintenance, and a quick one-minute pick-me-up exercise. There are also guidelines in Chapter 5 for those who wish to carry their practice further.

The ailment section forms the bulk of the book. When you are unwell, you can take it out of your pocket or handbag, even while in the office, or while traveling; you can look up your health problem in the alphabetical listings, and get instantaneous help—by using the affirmations and color visualizations, and by stimulating the relevant pressure points—to treat any ailment, there and then.

Color Zone Therapy can influence your daily life, and your mental and physical health, by just using the energy sources that nature has made available to all of us. In this book you will learn to use and focus your energy to best help others and yourself. You will learn to help your body and your glands to function at 100 per cent of their capabilities, maintaining a feeling of youth, vigor, enterprise and energy. You will need to have perseverance, love, belief and, above all, unshakable faith; but the opportunity is there for you to seize. If you make Color Zone Therapy part of your everyday routine, you will find it to be a very big winner.

Joseph Corvo &
Lilian Verner-Bonds

Introducing Color Zone Therapy

WHAT IS COLOR ZONE THERAPY?

COLOR ZONE THERAPY combines two dynamic thera-pies—Zone Therapy and Color Therapy. Zone Therapy is a form of treatment, grounded in medical science, which uses stim-ulation of specific key points on the feet, hands and face to treat the whole physical system of the body via the glands and internal organs. In this book, we will focus mainly on treatment using the feet. There is some correlation between the thinking behind reflex-ology and Zone Therapy, but reflexology is only one aspect of zone work. The specifics of Zone Therapy are discussed in Chapter 2. Joseph Corvo has really put Zone Therapy on the map with his best-selling books and videos, seminars and television appearances.

Color Therapy is an approach that has been used since the earliest of times, and which is currently expanding in recognition by leaps and bounds. Color is used comprehensively as a key to the whole process of assessing a person's condition, discovering the underlying causes of health problems, and putting treatment into practice. Lilian Verner-Bonds has developed her own meth-ods in this field through her private practice and workshops, finding a unique way of extending the benefits beyond physical health, into the realms of mental, emotional and spiritual well-being. This is described in depth in Chapter 3.

ABOUT THE AUTHORS

Joseph Corvo is a born healer and has been a Zone Therapy practitioner for 37 years. From the age of four, he was aware that he could see things other people could not see. Later on he became aware that he was gifted with second sight. By the time he was seven, he was healing on a regular basis. By laying on of hands, he found he could achieve amazing results.

At the age of 14, Joseph started work down a coal mine. However, he was blessed with a completely natural voice and his musical ability enabled him to leave the pit and start a career as a singer. He studied voice and opera in Rome and successfully became an operatic tenor.

In America, he met Franz Heubach, a disciple of the great Dr William Fitzgerald, the discoverer of Zone Therapy. He was invited by Heubach to study Zone Therapy and has since gone on to become a master of the technique. Joseph's reputation has spread worldwide and he is known as "the Miracle Worker". His books have sold in 26 countries and his client list reads like *Who's Who*. He has dedicated himself to the therapy, which he describes as the "most original procedure in medicine today".

Lilian Verner-Bonds is a leading clairvoyant color healer, and an international lecturer, teacher and author. Even before Lilian was five years old, her clairvoyant talents were becoming evident; during the Second World War, while hiding in London bomb shelters, she discovered she could read palms, managing to find out all she needed to know about a person from holding their hands, when it was impossible to talk during the noise of a raid.

In 1984, after a successful theatrical and television career, Lilian decided to give up acting in order to pursue her personal quest. Some time before, she had experienced a voice telling her that she should now begin to work not in the spotlight, but with a different kind of light—the supreme light whence all color comes. She began in-depth studies of counseling and personal growth methods and color in relation to health. She found that she was able to harness her ability with clairvoyance, combine it with this knowledge, and channel it into Color Therapy for use in health and healing. She spent fourteen years in a developing psychic circle, and also learned shiatsu. Realizing the enormous power of color as what she now calls the "great corrective", she set up her private practice in 1984.

Over the years, Lilian has developed her own unique

technique of "color relating", which enables her to assess the state of an individual's wellbeing—physical, mental and emotional. This process reveals anyone's patterns of the past and present, as well as their current direction for the future; it can reveal why they may not be getting what they want from life. Lilian then uses color counseling to help them restore the lost balance. She has further developed her work in color psychology with the use of chromotherapy, which is the art of physically exposing the individual to correctly chosen colored light in order to deal with their specific issues of health and wellness. She has an extremely busy practice, with many prominent clients, and is author of a book and tape, both published worldwide, on the subject.

HOW COLOR ZONE THERAPY CAME ABOUT

We first met six years ago, when introduced by a client who had been helped by, and was enthusiastic about, both our methods of healing. As we talked about our apparently quite distinct methods, we immediately began to realize that there was in fact a fundamental sense of connection between them. On the one hand, there were strong common elements and areas of overlap, and at the same time there was evident an extraordinary complementarity. That is to say, we quickly realized that our two forms of therapy each supply to one another the elements that together create a comprehensive whole, a broader overall approach that truly offers a complete approach to achieving Total Health. To us Total Health is the result of the totality of the aspects of how you live and what you do; it is more than immediate physical wellbeing—this totality is often described in terms of mind, body and spirit. In our work we help people to become well and stay well, to experience wellness in the whole of their person. We each experienced the sense that the other's approach actually represented what we had already been intuitively adding to our own discipline for years in order to broaden its possibilities.

How the combination works

The connection between our two approaches works in the following way. All three of our "bodies", physical, mental and emotional, are manifestations of the working of electromagnetic energy—the fundamental stuff of life, the vibrations of which even solid matter is composed. For complete health, this energy must flow unimpeded through all three of these systems.

We know from science that the body is an electromagnetic field, with currents constantly flowing through it. Ten main currents run through the body, aligned respectively with the toes and fingers, and the area covered by each current is termed a *zone*, with five zones on each side of the body. All organs, glands and elements of the nervous system fall into these zones.

Zone Therapy and Color Therapy both work with the flow of electromagnetic energy, and complement one another in their ways of working to improve this flow. Zone Therapy uses physical stimulus, while Color Therapy works through more intangible stimuli, ie the emotions. But both of us had been incorporating in our work, for years, the conviction that the diseases and illnesses that prove most difficult to cure manifest because of those underlying mental and emotional attitudes. Joseph, in fact, was already using color informally in his work, and Lilian had been incorporating pressure-point techniques adapted from shiatsu. Both of us had also, in fact, been working as healers since childhood, and both of us are motivated by a higher force that we see as the vital source for promoting health and relieving suffering.

We were stunned by this discovery, and immediately began to work together on patients' cases, and also on joint teaching. Out of some years of this cooperative working has evolved a broader approach, a continued fusing and integrating of methods, which has been further developed and refined into the contents of the book you now hold in your hands. The comprehensive approach to identifying and replacing specific negative attitudes and thought patterns is a core element. The resulting method of Color Zone Therapy is truly able to inspire the desire and determination, the positivity and will, that enables achievement of true health and happiness for everyone, instantly.

COLOR ZONE THERAPY IN ACTION—
CASE HISTORIES

Color Zone Therapy really can change your life. Below, Lilian relates some case histories, showing how this has come about for some of our clients. These case histories show how we use our method in practice, dealing with some serious but still common-place ailments—severe back problems, childhood asthma and chronic addiction. The patients' names have been changed in the interests of confidentiality.

Jennie's story

Jennie came to see Joseph and me a few years ago. She was sitting before us on the healing couch in the treatment room. She was overweight and clearly in pain; it had been difficult for her even to get on to the couch.

Jennie explained that she was an assistant to a high-profile executive. Four years ago, she said, she had been involved in a car crash and had sustained a severe back injury. Since that time she had been in constant, chronic pain; every treatment she had tried had failed to help.

"I just cannot bear any more of this pain," Jennie said. Her voice was desperate. "And it's worst of all when I am sitting at my desk in the office. I told my boss that I would have to give up work, and he said that I had to come and see you. And I've put on extra weight. Quite frankly, you're my only hope."

"Please lie still, now, Jennie," I said to her, as Joseph sat beside her feet, with his customary start to the process. "Start to relax; breathe very slowly and deeply. Now, I want you to imagine that the top of your head can open, and that a beautiful beam of indigo colored light is pouring down into your body from above. And I want you to picture that, as this rich, deep blue light flows into you, a million silver stars are cascading around you and off into the air, sparkling and bubbly. Each of these stars matches one of the tears that you have been shedding in your suffering. And now, this blue light turns into a warm liquid which gently seeps down your spine, bathing and soaking each vertebra in its healing vibration."

Jennie was now in a deep, meditative state, gently trembling with the energies of the color. Meanwhile, Joseph quietly took her right foot. Holding it firmly in one hand, he prepared to use just one finger of the other hand to apply pressure at a single spot—a point on the sole, towards the heel and on the inside edge of the foot—which relates to the lower back and spinal column. He pressed just once, with a sharp movement, and then sat back. Jennie immediately gasped, and her eyes flew open. "My God!" she cried, "I just felt a bolt of lightning shoot through my leg and hit me in the back, right in the spot where the pain is!"

"Close your eyes," I continued. "Now you can relax again, and feel the opening at the top of your head closing. But allow the color to remain with you for a little longer, and continue to breathe deeply." Jennie lay still.

"Come on, now," said Joseph after a few minutes. "You're OK; off you go." Jennie gingerly sat up and lowered her legs on to the floor. Suddenly she burst into tears. "It doesn't hurt any more!", she cried, "It doesn't hurt! I can't believe it. This is the first time in four years that I've been free of pain!"

Two years later, Joseph and I were at a reception when this beautiful, slim lady sidled up to us. "Do you remember me?" she said. "I'm the fat lady who came to see you with the back problem. Well, since your treatment, I've not had the pain again—and within nine months the extra weight had all dropped off me. It's been a miracle. I've been able to continue in my position at work, and my life has returned to normal. Thank you so much."

Timmy's story

Timmy was fifteen years of age, and suffered from chronic asthma; he arrived for treatment with his mother. Joseph and

I decided to see them together, for the benefit of Timmy's healing. In asthma, there is often a deep subconscious underlying motive that life is altogether too much of a burden for the sufferer. Physically, this manifests as a rejection of present life situation, by means of the bronchial tubes simply refusing to work any more; they quite literally collapse under the strain. In children, there can also be an unhealthy attachment to the mother's problems. In other words, the mother's anxieties are picked up by the child— even though this may be the very last thing the mother wants for her child; these are the typical dynamics of the situation.

Timmy lay on the couch. I asked him to take several deep breaths in and out, to begin to relax, and at the same time to imagine the top of his head opening to allow a beautiful beam of bright orange light to pour straight down into his chest. Timmy's mother was sitting nearby, watching intently.

I continued: "The light is very warm and relaxing now Timmy; and as it goes down into your chest, it turns into a soft, cool liquid and gently pushes its way into the little tubes in your lungs, making each of them open widely, and become calm." At this point, Joseph took Timmy's right foot; he focused especially on the area relating to the lungs and bronchi, under the fourth toe. He then proceeded to the points for the thyroid and pituitary glands, then for the nervous system, the thymus gland, and the prostate.

"Now, I want you to repeat this after me," I said, "I don't have to give up myself to please others; I am free to do what I want." This is a *positive replacement affirmation*, which I asked Timmy to keep on repeating. Meanwhile, Joseph worked in the same way on both Timmy's feet; at the same time his head was bent over them, as he concentrated healing power through his hands. The whole treatment lasted twenty minutes, with Timmy still pulling the orange light into his lungs, and repeating to himself the affirmation.

I then asked Timmy to close the opening in his head, to remember the orange light filling his lungs and to repeat the healing lines once more. Joseph closed his hands over both feet for one minute longer. "There, that's done now," he said. "You can go home." Timmy went out to the reception room, while his mother remained. Tears began to stream down her face. "I've had such a hard time for years now," she said, "my husband goes away to work at sea for such long periods. I have to take care of the family on my own. I had to give up my job as a nurse to take care of them all, and it's been a lonely struggle. So Timmy has to be the man of the house.

"Sitting here with Timmy, just now," she went on, "I imagined that orange light going down into my chest too, I felt a great surge of heat from it. It gave me an extraordinary sense of comfort and strength. I just don't seem to be afraid any more."

Before Timmy and his mother left, Joseph showed them how to do the treatment themselves on the feet, and also how to apply pressure to the floor of the mouth, underneath the root of the tongue, and to the tongue itself. These points all need to be worked on for the relief of asthma, for they free the blockages that asthma creates around the corresponding organs (you will find details of how to do this yourself in Chapter 2).

Timmy's mother had revealed a classic reason for Timmy's distress—he had unwittingly been taking on a father's role, far beyond his years, and had dovetailed this perfectly with his mother's problems by giving her something to "nurse" at home, which would thus replace her lost career. This is exactly the sort of unspoken agenda that goes on in very many families.

Timmy has never needed to return for treatment; he has not even had an asthma attack since then. His mother telephones from time to time, to give a report on his progress. "It seems to have done the trick," she says. "It's just fantastic! He can play football with his friends now. Thank you!" The situation of Timmy and his mom is clearly one where both mother and child were able to heal themselves through the same process, at the same time.

Douglas' story

Douglas was lying on the couch; he was in his late sixties, and led a very high-profile social life. He had been one of Joseph's patients for a number of years. Joseph had successfully treated his arthritis in the hip and shoulders, but Douglas was also an alcoholic. Joseph had realized that this was at the root of his problems, and that the emotional aspect of the problem required treatment, so he had called me in too.

Joseph sat on the couch, took one of Douglas's feet in his hands, and began to gently massage and stimulate the points relating to the adrenal glands. "Douglas," I said, "Please close your eyes, relax, and take deep in and out breaths. Now, imagine an opening in the top of your head, and a stream of beautiful indigo light pouring into it from above; feel this color filling your whole body."

Douglas imagined this, while Joseph continued to work silently on his feet. I went on: "Tell me about your day, Douglas. What would you say is the highlight of your day?"

"I think that would be at six o'clock, when I relax and have my first gin and tonic."

"And how many of those do you have, Douglas?"

"Well, it depends...". He paused, then continued, laughing: "Mother always had her pre-drinks, every evening, so I suppose I just followed suit. It seemed to be fun."

"Douglas, I want you to imagine that you have a drink in your hand—a gin and tonic. You are now lifting it to your lips. Can you see that drink, Douglas?"

"Yes, I can," he said.

"Look at that drink. Stare at it. Now I want you to be aware, as you look at that drink, that you have to make a decision. You have a choice—it's either this liquor, or it's your life." Silence followed for about a minute. Then Douglas's eyes suddenly flew wide open. He sat bolt upright, as though he had just received a shock.

"I'd never thought of it like that before," he uttered; his face wore a startled expression. Then he began repeating the affirmation over and over again, "It's the liquor or my life; the liquor or my life...". Joseph had now treated additional points for liver, kidney, pancreas, thymus gland, pituitary gland, thyroids and nervous system, on both feet. He withdrew his hands.

"Close your eyes, Douglas," I said. "Imagine closing the top of your head, and relax. You are free now."

Douglas did not return for further treatments—he hasn't needed to. He hasn't touched a drop of alcohol since that day. "I can't understand it," he commented to Joseph and me, some time later, "I don't even have the desire to drink. It's a miracle."

PUTTING IT INTO PRACTICE

In Chapters 2 and 3, we will tell you more about the workings of Zone Therapy and Color Therapy, before going on to show how to put Color Zone Therapy into practice for yourself in Chapter 4.

2

The Principles of Zone Therapy

ZONE THERAPY is as old as the human race. All your life you have used it without knowing it. If you have toothache, what do you do? You automatically put your hand to your jaw for comfort. If you have a headache, the first thing you do is to place your hand on the affected part of your head—and notice that you do it firmly. You do this because you have discovered that the pressure eases the pain. When you go to the dentist, you grip the chair as hard as possible and stiffen yourself, for the same reason. You have this unconscious knowledge that pressure eases pain. You intuitively know that there is virtue in pressure, if you only knew precisely how to apply it.

Some people will try to tell you that Zone Therapy was discovered by some guru sitting on the top of a mountain, but this is not true. Zone Therapy was discovered by Dr William Fitzgerald of Hartford, Connecticut, in the early part of this century. He was a graduate of the University of Vermont, and he spent two-and-a-half years in the Boston City Hospital. He served two years in the London Central Nose and Throat Hospital in England and two years in Vienna, where he was assistant to Professors Politzer and Chiari. For several years Dr Fitzgerald was senior nose and throat surgeon of St Francis Hospital, Hartford, Connecticut.

As stated in Chapter 1, Zone Therapy is a unique, medically orientated system, grounded in medical science and a natural adjunct to conventional medicine. We also mentioned that the body is an electromagnetic field, with invisible electrical currents running through ten zones in line with the fingers and toes—five on each side of the body—and covering all the organs, glands and nervous systems.

Toxic poisoning is an aspect of very many diseases and conditions of ill-health. The theory of Zone Therapy is that because of the toxic substances we are exposed to in our food and drink or in the air we breathe, harmful crystalline deposits form at the nerve endings, and these deposits keep the electrical contact or impulse from grounding, thus interfering with the flow of electromagnetic currents around the body. Aging and illness occur because the balance of the electromagnetic field is upset—if only minimum power is flowing through a zone, the glands or organs in that zone will start to deteriorate quickly. Zone Therapy therefore employs prolonged pressure to points on the soles of the feet (or hands) which relate to the various parts of the body, in order to clear congestion from the area. If the congestion is very deep, the point of pain referral on the foot or hand will feel sore. Stimulating this point produces a counter-irritation, which is referred to the problem areas within the body; and it is this which gives relief, detoxification and healing.

The distinction between Zone Therapy and foot reflexology, mentioned in Chapter 1, is of interest here. Zone Therapy is actually the mother of reflexology. Dr William Fitzgerald was the master of this whole approach to working on the whole body, and called it Zone Therapy; Eunice Ingham in New York and Dr Joe Reilly then took up part of this approach, focusing on the feet, and developed it into reflexology, which is thus an offshoot of zone work.

You *are* your glands and organs, so any malfunction in these leads to poor health. Keep your glands and organs free of congestion and toxins, and you will achieve good health. The glands and organs can't function properly and process waste products if they are congested. Each needs to be functioning well, otherwise it affects the balance of the others. It can be said that most complaints are caused through lack of nourishment through glands and organs.

Zone Therapy not only relieves pain; it will remove the cause of the pain and, if persisted with, will clear up all the associated difficulties being experienced within the body. Zone Therapy has already worked for a million people, and it will work for you. Zone Therapy will eventually become as natural to you as brushing your teeth, for yourself and for your family.

You cannot injure yourself in any way using Zone Therapy. The system is perfectly safe and is simplicity itself, yet the technique must be carried out in an exact manner. It cannot be done haphazardly. Specific instructions will be given in Chapter 4 for a variety of different ailments or health problems.

THE TEN BODY ZONES

Zone One

Goes from the tip of the thumb straight up to the top of the head and down through the nostril to the big toe. The main part of the stomach lies in the first zone, as well as uterus, bladder, vagina or prostate.

Zone Two

Goes from the index finger to the head and straight down to the second toe.

Zone Three

Goes from the second finger up to the head, and down to the third toe. The appendix is in zone three, on the right side.

Zone Four

Goes from the fourth finger up to the head and down to the fourth toe.

Zone Five

Goes from the little finger up to the head and down to the little toe.

Other glands and organs

The first, second and third zones on the left side of the body include the heart and pancreas.

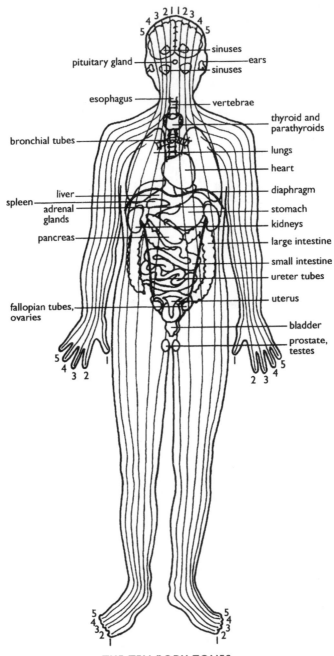

pituitary gland

esophagus

bronchial tubes

spleen
liver
adrenal
glands
pancreas

fallopian tubes,
ovaries

5
4
3 2

sinuses

ears

sinuses

vertebrae

thyroid and
parathyroids

lungs

heart

diaphragm

stomach

kidneys

large intestine

small intestine

ureter tubes

uterus

bladder

prostate,
testes

1

1

2 3

5
4

THE TEN BODY ZONES

The eyes, ears, sinuses, bronchial tubes and lungs are in the second and third zones, as well as the liver (on the left side of body). The kidneys are in the third and fourth zones, on either side.

THE GLANDS

As well as the major organs, the glands are extremely important in Zone Therapy. As their functioning is not as well known as that of the major organs, here is a brief introduction to what they do and why their treatment is vital in almost all ailments.

Glands are organs that form and release hormones—substances that act elsewhere in the body, in order to aid regular functions such as perspiration, digestion or immunity and resistance to infection. Some of these substances are carried in the blood, and others go directly to the surface of the skin, or to the lining of an organ such as the stomach.

The pituitary gland

The pituitary is the master gland, the most complex of the glands that work through the blood flow. It produces a number of hormones with a variety of purposes, including stimulating the adrenal glands, the thyroid glands, the ovaries or testes, the control of growth, birth labor and the secretion of mother's milk, pigment in the skin, and water retention. It is located in the bottom of the skull, with the upper part at the base of the brain, and the lower part in the roof of the mouth. If there is an imbalance in the pituitary, all the above functions will begin to suffer, especially the functioning of the thyroid and adrenal glands, and eventually other organs will begin to malfunction—notably the pancreas, liver and kidneys.

The thyroid gland

The thyroid produces thyroxine, which is released into the bloodstream to accelerate the release of energy into the body tissues from the combustion of glucose, allowing an increase in the rates of bodily and mental activity, and of breathing and blood

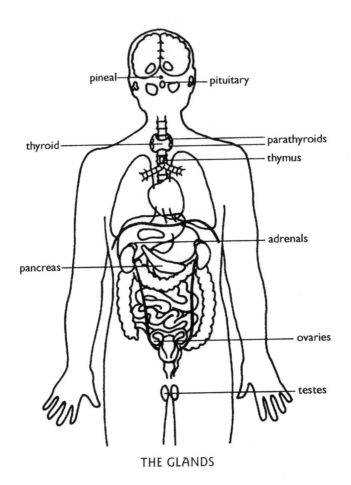

THE GLANDS

circulation by the heart to meet added demands for oxygen. The thyroid is also the main store for iodine in the body. It is located in the front of the neck, around the windpipe, on either side of the Adam's apple. Although it lies near the surface, it is small and soft and can scarcely be felt, provided it is in a healthy state.

If there is a lack of iodine in the body, the supply of thyroxine will be insufficient; the body metabolism will slow down, together with blood circulation and breathing. Digestion will also be hindered, and constipation experienced; there will be a general shortage of energy and vitality, with weight gain. Other effects include loss of memory, unstable menstruation, dry and scaly skin, loss of hair and hair quality, and distress and low spirits.

The parathyroid glands

These are four small glands embedded behind the thyroid. They produce parathormone, which regulates the concentration of calcium and phosphorus in the blood. Calcium is required not only for growth and replacement of bones and other tissue, but also for the nerves and to enable muscles to relax. If these glands malfunction and too much parathormone is produced, too much calcium can be withdrawn from the bones to maintain blood calcium level, resulting in osteoporosis, which makes the bones increasingly fragile. The surplus calcium in the blood is then excreted in the urine and may form kidney stones. Another aspect of parathyroid malfunctioning is nervousness and over-excitability, with rapid beating of the heart.

The thymus gland

This is located at the root of the neck, and mainly lies below the top of the sternum or breastbone. It consists mostly of developing white blood cells, which are concerned with immunity to infection. In conventional medical opinion, the thymus is considered only really to be of importance in infancy and early childhood (after which it stops growing), considering that it can be removed in later life without effect. In infancy, it enables the development of immunity to infectious microbes, and causes the body to reject proteins other than its own, thus accounting for allergic reactions and rejection of transplanted organs. Auto-immune diseases (such as AIDS) relate very strongly to the condition of this gland, and serious disorders will advance more strongly if the thymus is in a weak state.

I believe that the thymus is perhaps of central importance among the glands. Emotional states such as shock, distress and even plain unhappiness are very much connected with it; bad news or grief will have an immediately adverse effect on it. Conversely, the ability to maintain positivity will have a beneficial effect on it, which will in turn enable the whole body to deal better with any incipient illness, and maintain general wellbeing.

The adrenal glands

These are a pair of small organs at the back of the abdomen, against the upper ends of the two kidneys. Known as the glands of fight-or-flight, they release minute amounts of the powerful hormone adrenalin (for instance, when we experience fear or anger) which diverts significant amounts of blood from skin and digestive organs to muscles, increasing the action of the heart, increasing blood pressure, releasing glucose as ready-for-action fuel for the muscles into the bloodstream, and slowing down digestion. The other function of the adrenals is the production of cortisol and aldosterone, which directly or indirectly influence a great many chemical processes in the body, serving to maintain a stable chemical status quo in the stresses of an ever-changing environment. Specific effects include the suppression of inflammation and the effects of allergy, the distribution of fat in the body, control of salt and water loss by the kidneys, maintaining the balance of sodium and potassium, on which the activity of muscle depends, and a degree of regulation of the sex hormones. More broadly speaking, without the benefit of these glands, such stresses as illness, injury, mental strain and severe exertion would actually be lethal to us.

The pancreas

This is at the back of the abdomen, near the stomach. As well as being an offshoot of the intestine, it is primarily important as a gland that controls digestion, producing the two hormones insulin and glucagon, which are released directly into the bloodstream and work together for the chemical control of sugar in the body, for storage or use in combustion to create energy for all mental and physical activity. Milder malfunctioning of the pancreas produces irregular blood sugar and thus wildly fluctuating energy levels, while diabetes represents the more serious effect.

The gonads

The gonads are the primary sex organs, in other words the ovaries in women and the testes in men. They excrete the sex hormones, which not only affect such important issues as sex drive, sexual health and reproductive functioning, but are also closely interconnected with the health of other organs including the pituitary, thyroid and adrenals, and the kidney, bladder and prostate.

Note

When consulting Chapter 4 about how to treat specific ailments, you may find it helpful to refer back to this section, so that you will understand exactly the benefits that the stimulation of the points for these glands is bringing you.

HOW TO PERFORM ZONE THERAPY

Prolonged pressure is applied to the areas on the soles of the feet that correspond to the parts of the body where problems lie (see diagrams on pages 22–23); these are also the areas where you will feel pain when you press. Later sections of the book will tell you which these will be for each ailment. Problems like corns and bunions cause a lot of trouble because they block off the nerve flow through that particular zone, thus causing trouble in the back and neck areas; if you suffer from these, it will be beneficial to go to a chiropodist for treatment, so that Zone Therapy work will be more effective. After chiropody, treat the affected areas gently. Pressure can sometimes be applied to other parts of the body, including the hands and tongue, but here we will mainly concentrate on the feet.

Hold your foot firmly with one hand and use the other hand to apply pressure—the more the pressure, the quicker the results seem to be; in fact it can be quite painful to those suffering from disease symptoms, until all the crystalline deposits have been broken down by a series of treatments. Pressure is applied with the top joint of the thumb or the middle finger. Make sure that your nails are cut short. If firmer pressure is required, or your fingers are weak, you can use a knuckle or the handle of a toothbrush. Other forms of treatment such as rolling the feet over a golf ball can also be very effective.

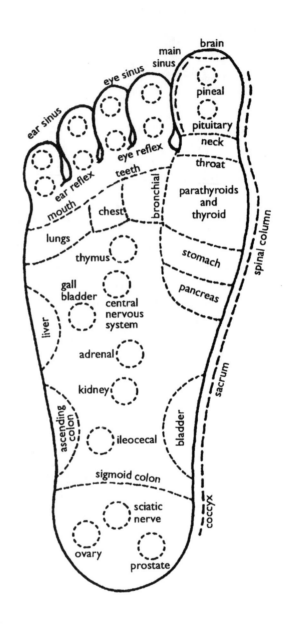

PRESSURE POINTS—RIGHT FOOT (SOLE)

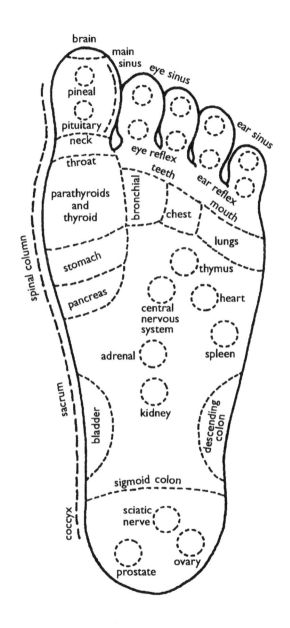

PRESSURE POINTS—LEFT FOOT (SOLE)

23

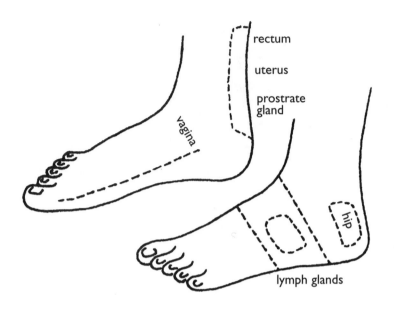

**PRESSURE POINTS ON
TOP OF FEET AND SIDE OF ANKLES**

Place the underside of your thumb on the area or point you are treating; put pressure on and rotate in an anti-clockwise motion. Press as deep as you can; work for five to ten seconds, then move to the next point you need to treat. Go to each point in rotation, eventually arriving back at the number one spot. Keep working over all the areas listed for your problem, working to eliminate the sore areas; give each foot five minutes. On occasion, the treatment for an ailment will suggest that you treat part of the hand or perhaps the tongue instead, because that is more effective for one or two conditions, such as asthma or menstrual problems. Detailed instructions will be given when required. The diagrams opposite show the locations of the points on the hands.

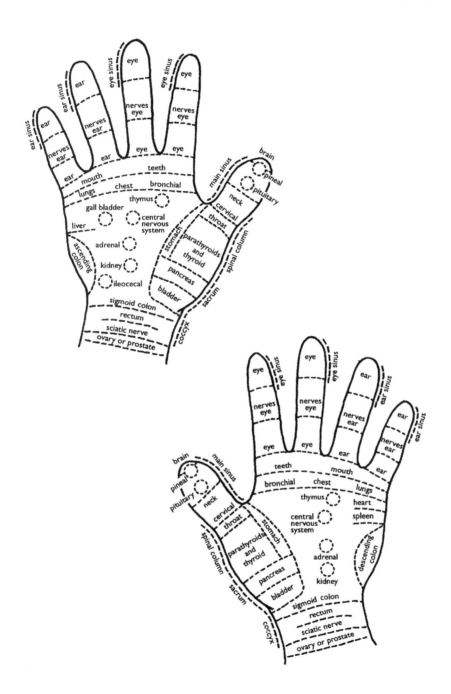

PRESSURE POINTS—THE HANDS (PALMS)

Working in this way will break down all the crystalline deposits which are choking and blocking all the nerve endings. After a series of treatments, with patience and determination, the deposits will disappear and you will feel infinitely better. Do not overdo the work in any zone. If you are not getting results, wait and try again later on.

EXERCISE

Try it now. Wear loose clothing, and sit in a comfortable position, where you can reach one foot at a time, and away from drafts. Apply pressure with your thumb or fingers over a variety of points on the feet. Start gently, and then go deeper until you feel some pain or soreness. Put on as much pressure as you can, and go as deep as you can comfortably bear. Notice how sensitive different points feel; if there is deep congestion, it can be very painful.

Now try a simple exercise for the treatment of fatigue. Referring to the diagram below, press, with the thumb or fingers, the points for the main gland that is relevant here, the thyroid. Then switch to the point for the adrenal gland, then the pituitary gland, then for the liver and finally back to the thyroid point. Do all this on one foot and then the other, for five minutes apiece. Drink a glass of water when you have finished. Because you are aiding detoxification, it is always beneficial to drink plenty of pure water in conjunction with the treatment.

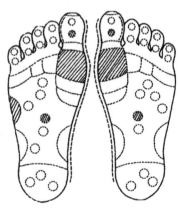

The best form of treatment would be twice a day, doing a ten-minute treatment (five minutes on each foot) night and morning. If you do not immediately contact the right zone, try the adjoining zones in the area. In working any zone for a specific trouble, you will also clear up any other conditions in that zone. The general pattern will be to work on the specific points for your particular condition, and then go on to give a general treatment to the points for all glands and organs. You could treat each of these for ten seconds, working systematically round all the points shown on the diagrams on pages 22–23.

Chapter 4 describes in detail how to use Zone Treatment in the combined form of Color Zone Therapy, and how to apply this for every common ailment.

Above all, be determined to succeed with the treatment.

3

The Principles of Color Therapy

COLOR can reveal the significance in our actions that cannot otherwise be revealed. This chapter is given over to exploring the meaning of color, both mentally, emotionally and physically. Color surrounds and affects everyone—and most of us take it for granted. But it is important that you have an understanding of the characteristics and nature of the seven colors of the rainbow.

We react to color automatically. Color healing is a wonderfully direct way of working on the body. Neither flesh, nor mental attitude, nor emotion is a barrier to color. Color is a gift of evolution. It influences our thoughts and social behavior, our health, our relationships; in fact we cannot live without the light which contains all color. If you put a plant in a cupboard and shut out the light it withers and dies. Even people without sight can sense the vibrations of different colors.

Color can be measured. All organs and parts of our bodies hold to a particular set of harmonious vibrations when they are healthy. Each organ has its own particular color and as such there will be a color that can heal it. Scientific research carried out in controlled environments, including mental homes and prisons, has shown that color has a measurable effect on the psychic and physical make-up of human beings.

Color comes from pure light. The clear light that holds all color is the clear brilliance from the sun. So color transcends the solid form. It is a glimpse into the infinite. When the light of the sun and stars reaches the earth, the colors of the spectrum break out of its brilliance. It's just like birth. Color will always bring you back into balance. It is the great corrective. When we are truly well, all the colors shine out from us in an ever-changing but always rhythmically serene light show.

Reading this chapter on color will encourage you to have a greater awareness of its nature. Then you can learn to appreciate and understand what it's saying to you, and how to use it for your own benefit on all levels.

Each color has many meanings; it influences our thoughts, our social behavior, our health and our relationships. If you learn its language, color has the ability to tell you how it really is for you because color is a problem-solver. It gives you information that allows you to color yourself healthy, wealthy and wise. Color has its codes and, because it is an intimate part of our being, it can point the way to bring order out of chaos.

From the psychology of color, we understand that every color has both positive and negative traits. Even the negative can be very positive, as this gives us clues about what needs attention. When a color has black in it, which makes it darker, it is called a shade, and it means that the color is on hold, or that the person's thoughts will be depressed. If the color has white in it, which makes it paler, it is called a tint; and the lighter the color gets, the more powerful the aspects of that color will be in force. All colors can have darker shades and lighter tints—an example would be the basic hue of red, which can become dark maroon or go to the other end of the scale and become pale pink. For the purposes of this book, I have kept to the basic seven colors of the spectrum or rainbow.

Each color section described later in this chapter will give you an overall understanding of the general qualities and characteristics of that hue. Remember, color is experienced directly. It is a vibration that will be felt in the body. Just as you use zone stimulation so you can use color to stimulate your system as well.

THE IMPORTANCE OF EMOTION

The spiritual body is probably the most commonly neglected component in the equation for Total Health. Yet it is arguably the most important element of all; it is our direct link with the universal intelligence and energy. It is this divine power that humankind experiences on earth through our emotions, which in turn affects our physical experience. It is our way of connecting with this force that is the real key to our success or failure at the most fundamental level.

COLOR AND EMOTION IN THE TREATMENT CHARTS

Each treatment chart for particular health problems, given in Chapter 4, gives the major color that treats that condition. If we were using Color Therapy only, several colors could be employed in conjunction with each other, but for this chart we focus on the principal color related to the problem.

For each ailment listed there is a section called "Underlying negative mental and emotional attitude"; it gives some understanding of what we are thinking in our deep subconscious—parts of our lives that we are not aware of—which is fueling our disease or complaint. Everything that happens to us in our lives has a mental thought pattern behind it. Some patterns are good for us; some are not. Even thoughts and ideas are vibrations, and can be "unwell" just as the liver or pancreas, or any other part of the body, can be unwell. These negative thought patterns will produce problems in time, and we will experience dis-at-ease in our lives because of it. We will always manifest physically that which we are not looking at or resolving subconsciously. To avoid this, we must allow anything we put to the back of our minds to come to the surface. When you identify the negative thought, then you can eliminate it. By keeping the negative thought submerged, when it does appear consciously it is usually as an illness of one sort or another. This negative thinking can identify what often is the cause of the problem—it gives the root cause or the core at the heart of the matter. Diseases and ailments can be reversed by just simply reversing the mental patterns that keep the illness fuelled. The psychology of color can reveal these. It is possible that all our diseases have negative thoughts behind them. Our emotions play a great part in keeping our bodies healthy. A happy mind creates a harmonious body, free of complaints.

Being aware of the negative thought behind a particular ailment enables you to replace it with a positive one. This is listed under the heading "Positive permanent thinking replacement" for each ailment. You repeat the phrase over and over again to yourself, so that it obliterates and stamps out the negative thought behind your problem. It's called an affirmation. While repeating the positive thinking replacement lines, also visualize the color given for your condition; you will not only be working to remove the problem thoughts that are at the core of the symptoms, but also, by imagining the healing color, you will be working with the energy of permanent healing.

USING MULTIPLE COLORS FOR TREATMENT

You will also notice that each of the seven colors of the rainbow is used several times for different diseases and complaints. This is because all colors have many attributes and abilities, and can heal a wide variety of conditions. Each color is like a diamond with many facets, which can be harnessed and used. All you have to do is just concentrate on the facet of the color, as listed in the affirmation section under your particular ailment, to bring about the relief you wish and desire. The energy of the color will be sent through the thought process of the words. You may want to note that orange, green and purple consist of two colors: orange is made up of red and yellow; green is made up of yellow and blue; and purple is made up of red and blue. So when reading about the color purple, say, for Alzheimer's disease, read the red and blue sections as well. As one of Alzheimer's sufferers' beliefs is to have a desire always to be in control, the red in the purple will give the person security, which is why someone wants to control in the first place. The blue in the purple will help to bring in for the person the truth of the matter, which is that we can't always have our own way!

The understanding of the emotional energy charges that are revealed in the *Eliminate* and *Repeat* sections in Chapter 4 was developed by tuning in to the vibration of color. The color stimulation plus positive thinking to eliminate damaging thoughts is a most powerful combination to combat pain and illnesses on all levels. We know that conventional medicine can deal with troublesome physical problems, but unless you go further and change the inner thought that accompanies the disease, it could return again and again. You need to make the change emotionally, that affects you physically, before you can bring about complete healing. It's never too late to reverse negative patterns and ways of thinking. By learning the language of color, you will be able to appreciate the entire spectrum of meanings that the intelligence of light is giving you. By visualizing the color given for each treatment, you will open yourself up to the influence of that healing vibration. Let your imagination wander into the land of color.

THE COLORS

RED (The Stimulator)

The color red governs the gonads.

The red area in the body is associated primarily with the genitals and reproductive organs. So, the glands in the body connected to the color red are the testes and the ovaries, and all functions of sexuality. Since ancient times, primitive peoples regarded the color red as the life force and nature has used red to attract the opposite sex to ensure the continuation of the species. Red is nature's sexual signal. We flush when we are sexually aroused, and our lips go redder, which is why women wear lipstick—we are subconsciously imitating this primal state!

Red signals life's energy, the zest and driving force of creation. Psychologically, the color red has the power to promote growth or cause destruction. The red color is primal; it is the first color of life and also the first color of the rainbow. It roots us. It is the color of the bottom part of the body—the lower trunk. As you go up the body so you go up the spectrum of color, just the same as the rainbow.

Red is a strong detoxifier; it will help to get rid of rubbish and remove negativity from your life, your psyche and your body. The muscles which have the power to act are also a red concern. It eases stiff limbs and joints, particularly the legs. Red is also useful in cases of paralysis.

Red can also be helpful for anyone who keeps catching colds

or chills easily, or for someone needing warmth in the case of hypothermia. Red can also cauterize inflammatory conditions but, if used too much, it can irritate and aggravate again.

If you feel sluggish, or if you are dreading something that you have to do, just work on visualizing the red color to give you support.

Red encourages you if you are "backward in coming forward". Red has a thrust and drive that pushes you on to achieve greater things. Red represents pioneering people, perseverance and strength of will. It is linked to gratitude and promotes cheerfulness. It is a great stimulator.

Red removes negativity; it is the color of respect. It can also indicate that you are over-stimulated or under pressure, therefore red will aggravate the condition, and this can cause anger and temper. Red can also show that you are on overload in life—irritability will show itself here. Red puts you in the hot seat. It is the color of adventure. A short sharp exposure to red quickens things along. Red really likes to help and it can save you. It can rescue you from any situation, such as inner hopelessness. Red is also the color that vibrates in the blood—the circulation. It is a great pick-you-up if you are feeling depressed, tired or lethargic—you can be assured that red will overcome. Red starts joy bubbling up. Red will bring out your potential and tell you it's time to go for it—go for it now!

POSITIVE RED
Leader, tenacious, dynamic perseverance

NEGATIVE RED
Lustful, intolerant, cruel, the bully, warmonger

POLARITY
GROWTH↔DESTRUCTION

ORANGE (The Socializer)

The color orange governs the adrenals.

Orange is the area of the lower intestines, the abdomen and kidneys. The adrenal glands sit on top of the kidneys; they are known as the "fright, flight and fight" glands. When our safety is threatened, adrenalin is secreted into the bloodstream to get us moving swiftly out of danger.

Orange provokes change, but with the awareness that change for the sake of change is not necessarily change for the better. Orange is the great gatherer, it represents the fruits of the earth, the harvest of the sun. Orange is the color of activity, enthusiasm and freedom. It is a great color for putting your life together again; it is full of promise when all seems shattered. If you are in grief, divorced, bereaved or in shock of any kind, orange can bring you out of it.

The part of the body associated with orange is the gut, which deals with the assimilation of food. Are you getting all the nutrients and goodness you need from life, both physically and spiritually? The profound meaning of this is that all experiences do matter, however painful. Refusing to take your experiences into yourself stops the flow of the life processes. This is what is at the basis of anorexia. The orange color does also help to physically increase the appetite.

So orange as a healing color is useful for any intestinal disorders or bowel disturbances. It is also a healer for the kidneys and bladder. In the case of rape, serious accident or even divorce, use orange to disperse the shock. Orange is a good aid for menopause and male change of life, as it balances the hormones; it can also help with infertility. The orange color also clears away mucus or catarrh that may be in the system.

Orange stirs up dormant conditions and brings them out into the open. For instance, you may find that you are unable to move forward in life because you cannot bury the past, keeping you stuck. But by using the stimulation of orange you can gain the strength to face up to and then break through these blocks, and thus be able to knit together your freed self once again. Orange can also be used for mental breakdowns and for anyone who feels suicidal. Depression responds well to orange stimulation.

Orange can also reveal any hidden phobias you may have. It gives you support to fight against unknown fears. The common feeling of fear usually indicates a need for orange in the system.

The color orange is genial and optimistic. It is a very social color. Orange is very humorous, and offers good companionship. Orange broadens life and is very purposeful. Orange is the color to create opportunity. By having the orange vibration in your system you can be sure that when opportunity knocks you'll be ready.

Orange moves on. Orange is physical intuition—through our gut instincts, it links us to our intuition. When a person is working with the orange aspect within their system, they intuitively know what to do to or what is right, regardless of intellect. If you have access to that, you are indeed master of your own destiny.

POSITIVE ORANGE
Flamboyance, warm-hearted, generous, warm-natured

NEGATIVE ORANGE
Exhibitionist, sponging, misleading, leans on others, pessimistic

POLARITY
ACTIVITY↔LAZINESS

YELLOW (The Communicator)

The color yellow governs the pancreas gland.

The color yellow governs the solar plexus which includes the liver, gall bladder, spleen and middle stomach. This yellow area covers our digestive system. Yellow also affects the skin and nervous system.

Yellow is the great eliminator of the spectrum. It cleanses and removes toxic waste from the body. Elimination is the law of life and faulty elimination is the cause of the beginning of most

diseases. Yellow tones and cleanses the system. It relieves constipation, which subconsciously represents a holding on to the past,
a fear of letting go.

The yellow area of color consciousness is also good to work
with for the removal of cellulite—another source of stored-up
waste. The great weight-watcher is yellow as this color helps the
flow of liquids, promotes the flow of gastric juices from the
digestion as well as other bodily fluids such as perspiration, tears
or oedema. It also feeds the central nervous system; it is a good
color to keep your nerves strong. Yellow gets you talking, which
helps clear the mind and correct forgetfulness.

Yellow has an agility of mind; it helps you to absorb facts
quickly, giving clarity and precision of thought. Yellow unravels
and reveals; it leaves no stone unturned. It has a knack of pin-
pointing the deep issues—yellow is inquisitive. It helps you think
through difficulties and explore all avenues.

People with the characteristics of a yellow personality find
it very difficult to rest—one thing seems to lead to another and
they never get a break. The yellow area reveals how good you are
at getting your personal needs met; it is the color of your
powerhouse.

Yellow is connected to the tongue, because yellow just loves
words. Yellow believes the pen is mightier than the sword; fur-
thermore, those who use the pen live longer! On the negative
side, acidic yellow can bring forth the acid tongue.

Yellow enjoys networking—whether by jungle drum or telephone. When something is revealed to yellow it immediately
thinks of editing it for the public rather than feeling it for itself.
Gossip is yellow. It's a good idea to work on stimulating the yellow color when there is a lack of confidence or shyness, or a
deep-rooted psychological belief that "I'm not good enough".
Yellow brings laughter, fun and joy and lifts depression. It can
remove a jaundiced view of life.

Yellow transforms "I can't" into "I can". It's the laughter
color, laughter being the best tonic. Laughter is internal aero-
bics; it massages your organs. Give your organs a treat; the best
medicine is a merry heart.

Yellow is very broad-minded; it despises pettiness. Love has
no boundaries—neither does yellow. Yellow is very diplomatic—

full of self-control, style and sophistication. It is concentration, so use the yellow color to get some sharpness in your life. Yellow is the great reasoner; everything must have proof and add up. But yellow shouldn't be afraid to be compassionate and follow intuition. Yellow is the brightest color of all, so make sure to let the sunshine of yellow come into your life.

POSITIVE YELLOW
Mental agility, probing, tolerant, broad-minded

NEGATIVE YELLOW
Sarcastic, forgetful, stupid, intellectually rigid, chatterbox, critical

POLARITY
EXPANSION ←→ CONTRACTION

GREEN (The Producer)

The color green governs the thymus gland.

Green is the heart center, it also represents the chest, shoulders and the lower lungs. Green is the great harmonizer and balancer of the universe. Green is an emotional indicator—if a balance of green is not attained it can lead to pains of the heart, including envy and jealousy. Green has the ability to experience wholeness and love. It is the color of emotional relationships. As green helps us dispel negative feelings, green applied during stormy periods in relationships will calm and cool the emotions. Green gives direction, so it can be used when you are trying to make up your mind or your heart.

Green is the sanctuary, the gateway to freedom, the halfway house where the lesson of love needs to be learned in order to pass through. It is the color of bonding, a wonderful color to get rid of negative emotions and mental stress. It reduces over-stimulation and restores stability.

Green is the decision maker. It can also discriminate, so if you are ever wavering and indecisive, just close your eyes and visualize green. It is very productive, particularly in business. Highly practical, green knows the value of money and loves to collect possessions. Green is generous, the giver. Green is a great host, the improver for all, it brings comfort into the world. Green is everything in the garden that leads you down the stem of the flower to the root cause; thus it is the diagnostic color— green holds the key.

Green is made up of yellow and blue. The yellow part is the last color of the magnetic, hot side of the spectrum; and blue is the first part of the cool, electric side. The yellow clarifies and the blue brings wisdom. So, together, they help you to remember what you need to know. This is vital, because most of our physical and psychological illnesses result from events and conditions in our past.

Green is a lover of harmony and balance, as it is neither hot nor cold, active nor passive, acid nor alkaline. Green is the great beautician. It is the color of the great reformer, which brings about change. The green personality does not like to follow routes—it creates better ones when the old have failed. Green is a good color to give reassurance to children from neglected and disturbed environments. Hyperactive children also benefit from its calming effects, as green is soporific. Green is the color that deals with claustrophobia, as it adds space. Green says, "This is my space. I'm going to move so clear out of my way."

Green is excellent for healing heart ailments, both physically and emotionally. It soothes headaches, and relieves biliousness and liver complaints. It is a good detoxifier, and can help control blood pressure and nerves. Green is a tonic! Green is the color that blends with all, so it is a general healer. If anyone is experiencing an overload of any color, green can be applied to neutralize it.

Above all, green holds the key to the memory which unlocks the deep and hidden causes of our physical and psychological illnesses. It gives direction when you don't know what to do next. Green likes a fresh beginning and a new start.

BLUE (The Lover of Truth)

The color blue governs the thyroid and para-thyroid glands.

The color blue governs the thyroid and para-thyroid glands. Blue is the color of the present time—the Aquarian age. The Aquarian is the seeker of truth, who must go forward in truth, or he or she will go backwards out of fear. Blue combats fear.

Blue is the higher order of intelligence. A blue personality listens closely to what you have to say, and then plays it back to you. Blue reasons things out quietly and with integrity; ambassadors are blue. Blue doesn't like to draw attention to itself. Blue doesn't like to lie; honesty is a key blue trait, even if blue is afraid of it. If you want to get the truth of it in your life, just think blue.

Blue's wisdom is the antidote for an imagination run wild because blue is a safe haven. Writers are born with energy of the blue ray. A person drawn to blue can show that they long for a change—usually a change of situation. Blue will look first before it leaps—but it does leap.

Blue is communication by the voice, because blue belongs to the throat area, and is linked to the upper lungs, arms and base of the skull. Infections of this area are psychologically related to "talking inwards", in other words not speaking out or up for yourself, just as you cough because you have swallowed your thoughts and cannot trust yourself to speak up. Blue will help this by counteracting the fear of "spitting it out". People trapped in this syndrome need to learn the power of the spoken word—not so much to help others, but to help themselves. They need to understand that what you don't ask for, you rarely get. If you need a promotion at work, or just an extra cuddle from someone, don't forget to imagine blue—it will help you speak up for yourself and be heard. Stiff necks can benefit from blue as well. A stiff neck indicates rigidity of thought, a fear of going with the flow and of being flexible. Blue will help dissolve this fear.

Blue is useful for children's ailments, such as teething and ear infections, throat infections, and speech and vocal problems. These problems are often about the child having been unable to speak out from fear of the row that would follow or of the effects of parents" arguments. If children are unable to say how upset they are, their throats habitually tighten and become sore. The needy child is in the negative blue state, and needs to be encouraged to stand on his or her own two feet. Likewise, blue is good for the bed-wetting child and for adult incontinence.

Blue is the color for modern-day stress and anxiety; it can help bring down blood pressure. Introduce blue for the relief of pain—it cools inflammations, helps nose bleeds and internal bleeding, reduces the pain of sciatica and soothes stomach ulcers.

Blue is not a good color to use if you want to lose weight; it is too static, and definitely does not shift that "excess baggage". I have observed that many people who are overweight feel an attraction to blue—this is because negative blue aids and abets them in remaining just as they are; losing weight would bring unwelcome confrontations, conflict and change. Blue is associated with becoming a martyr, and with being stuck in a rut—the "doormat" syndrome.

The blue color represents peace with a purpose, fulfillment and contentment. Blue generally has a tranquil spirit, and is well balanced. It is the color to contemplate with, and makes you aware of the need to rest and relax.

Blue represents the acknowledgement of your family roots. It can show if there was a lack of values in your family. If you need to make a change in your life, use your highly inventive talents by bringing more blue into your life.

Blue sometimes feels manipulated by events, but it can also be the manipulator. When the blue areas in your body are unbalanced, you become emotionally upset, and this is liable to make things slide. Blue can then become very separate, even cold and snobbish; it can have a moody and unforgiving temperament.

True blue has a great quality of being able to "sober up". It brings a wisdom into love. Blue works in a discreet and tactful way. It prefers to maintain the status quo. It does not like confrontation and commotion. Blue does things with honor and sincerity, even if it doesn't always go by the book. Blue can penetrate the soul. It is the spiritual sedative. It has an acceptance of that which cannot be changed and it makes the best of what is. It has great belief that all will turn out right in the end. Blue is the spirit of truth. Go with the flow—the truth will always set you free.

POSITIVE BLUE
Truthful, patient, healer, integrity, spiritual
philosopher, teacher

NEGATIVE BLUE
Weak, emotionally unstable, spiteful, frigid, unforgiving

POLARITY
KNOWLEDGE←→IGNORANCE

INDIGO (The Spirit of Justice)

The color indigo governs the pituitary gland.

The pituitary is sometimes known as the conductor of the orchestra (the orchestra physically being the endocrine system). Indigo also represents the skeleton—the bones, particularly the backbone. The lower brain, the eyes and the sinuses are also related to indigo. The blue-black of indigo is the one color that can show up hidden fear, so look for a fear that you may not even know you have! One strange aspect of this is that indigo can show a very deep fear of fire. This is often related to an experience in a past life.

A positive aspect of indigo is that it can look beyond the complaint itself and get to the structure that caused the trouble. So, if you know there is something wrong and you can't quite put your finger on it, just imagine the indigo color and see what comes up. As you do this be aware of any emotions you may feel or sensations in the body. By working with this color you will also be strengthening the structure of your life and be providing a backbone of stamina to any endeavors you may have in mind.

Indigo is the strongest painkiller in the spectrum, and an antiseptic that can clear up any bacteria or the effects of pollution in air, water and food—as well as astral toxins (astral toxins are negative vibrations that we pick up in the psyche from the atmosphere and become lodged in the subconscious). Because the area of the ears, eyes and nose fall under its domain, indigo is good for acute sinus problems and cataracts. Experience shows that sinusitis and allied problems are very often the result of uncried tears from childhood.

Indigo is very good for lung and chest complaints, such as bronchitis and asthma, and for the treatment of lumbago, migraine, eczema, bruising and inflammations. Indigo can be used in short spells for the overactive thyroid, and also aids kidney complaints. It is a good color to work with to disperse growths, tumors and lumps of any kind. And, as indigo is said to promote tissue growth, it is also good for burns. Indigo is also the color for the back. Psychologically, backaches may indicate that we are holding ourselves back in life.

Indigo can show up addictions of any kind—drugs, alcohol, cigarettes. Addiction says, "There is something wrong with my life." Perhaps it has no structure or else the existing structure is not valid. This relates to us in our emotional lives and welfare, as well as at the physical level, as indigo represents the skeleton and bones in our bodies. Without a good spine, our bodies collapse and we can't stand up—just as our lives can't stand up if we are still being affected by a badly "constructed" childhood. Indigo always pares down to the bone. Thus indigo is also the great healer of painful memories. It helps a person to regain direction, after being emotionally shattered. It helps to prepare for the next step. As indigo is the spirit of perception, it will promote higher inspirational thoughts; it is the great purifier and purger. It is the "I wish" color, the opener of the third age. It clears out decay, so with it you can look to what you have to get rid of in life.

The indigo personality is very devoted, but this devotion is nearly always to work; indigo must be careful that work does not become the sole interest in life. Indigo is a lover of justice and is forever defending people's rights. The indigo personality will be conscientious and totally reliable in a crisis, but it must learn to surrender sometimes.

Indigo is a dramatic color—it has no in-betweens. There is a tendency to be up in the clouds one minute and down in the dumps the next. There is a great enthusiasm to start things and then drop them just as quickly. Indigo has also to be aware of self-deception and a desire to show off, which can make it unpopular. It must try to keep an unbiased outlook. But indigo is also the color that gets behind the cause of the trouble. This wonderful vibration will help to release you from imposed or self-acquired conditioning.

Indigo unravels the unknown. It has the ability to plan for the future. Indigo can see more than is seen. Indigo is very reverent. It loves tradition. Indigo has unshakable beliefs. It will uphold the establishment until the end. Indigo is law and order; it is the judge and jury.

Indigo's devotional aspect, combined with its reforming fervor, enables it to reconstruct organizations—religious and otherwise. Indigo must watch that devotion does not become its sole interest. Indigo will always hold the fort—it thinks it's indispensable—but it must learn to let someone else do it for a while. Indigo is a very dramatic color. The acting profession comes under the indigo ray.

Indigo is most powerful. On a spiritual level it says, "I see, I really do". Indigo will always work if there is a real need. It has the power of mind and thought with real understanding. It unravels the unknown.

PURPLE (The Mystic Leader)

The color purple governs the pineal gland.

Physically, purple represents the top of the head, the crown, the brain and the scalp. All mental orders relate to this ray. When employing purple for healing, it must be used carefully as it is a heavy color and too much of it can be depressive. Never work with this color if there is a history of depression or suicide. It is not a color recommended for use on young children, so if you really want to use it for a child, do so sparingly.

An overload of the purple vibration within the physical system can be detected by a person feeling isolated. If you have ever felt lonely or apart from life, just acknowledge your own individuality. You are a leader and this will always keep you apart from the crowd. Be assured that it is all right to march to the beat of a different drum. People who have a problem with purple are usually perfectionists. Purple can find itself going round and round in circles to find answers.

Purple is very useful for any kind of internal inflammation. It is very good for sciatica. It can also be the color to help skin eruptions subside. Purple is good for subduing palpitations of the heart. Purple can also help with any head and scalp problems and concussion. The immune system can also be given a boost with purple and it can soothe jangled nerves. Tired and sore eyes improve with the color purple. Purple is beneficial to help calm people who are emotionally erratic.

Purple is a powerful color; it is the peace maker. It combines power with gentleness. Purple sees a richness with quality on a very high level. When you are highly creative, you can be sure the purple areas in your body are well balanced. The purple personality prefers to be self-employed. Purple is always found in the corridors of power, it is always leader of the pack and will always be playing a prominent role in the community.

Purple is the great teacher who realizes that the pupil has to understand. Facts alone are not enough. Purple will sacrifice itself for the benefit of all without being a victim or a martyr. Purple is the color of great force. It shows direction. It has no limitations. It is the highest form of humanitarian—a very kind, lovable person. It combines power with gentleness, but its kindness will not be mistaken for weakness—it commands respect. Absorb the color purple to bring forth and acknowledge your hidden strengths and resolve to start using them from now on. If you feel lonely or apart from life and on the point of giving up, just bring the color purple into your imagination. Purple is the great protector.

As purple is a combination of red and blue it becomes a union of body and spirit—the visionary. Purple can see and feel things without using the physical senses. When the purple energy within us is working in a balanced way, purple uses its psychic perception on an everyday basis. This color produces the great mystical leader, combining humility with wisdom. Purple will make your inner candle burn bright. Purple is the heart of the universe in your hands.

POSITIVE PURPLE
Humanitarian, inventiveness, powerful orator, the protector

NEGATIVE PURPLE
Ruthless, corrupt, belligerent, treacherous,
pompous, arrogant

POLARITY
PEACE ←→ CONFLICT

Color Zone Therapy for Common Ailments

An A to Z of illnesses and their treatment

HOW TO USE THE CHARTS

FIRST FIND your health problem or ailment in the alphabetical section that follows these introductory pages.

Sit where you will be comfortable and warm, and able to reach your feet, unless someone else will be treating them for you. Wear loose clothing. Read up on the causes of your problems which are given under the heading "Underlying negative mental and emotional attitudes". This will give you clues as to the thoughts, at the back of your mind, that may be behind your condition. Then read up on the "Positive permanent thinking replacement". This is what you should use to replace the negative thought, by repeating it to yourself over and over again while you do your healing. This is an affirmation.

Beside the name of each disease you will notice that a "healing color" is given. This is the color that you should concentrate on while making the positive affirmation. If you find this difficult to do at first, just gaze at something that is the color you require. For instance, if you want to visualize the color green, just find a green apple and stare at it for one whole minute. Then close your eyes immediately, and continue to see that color, by remembering it visually. You can also imagine the top of your head opening and a beam of light pouring into it. Only use the color that is given in the chart.

At the end of each individual treatment chart is a diagram which will show you how to work on yourself physically with the Zone Therapy pressure points. The way to do this is explained in Chapter 2 (beginning on page 21) and you should study it carefully. The pressure points have been given to highlight the zone treatment for each particular complaint. In addition to this specific work, it is important, whenever possible, whatever your condition, also to work on the other glands and organs, so that they are all working at 100 percent. This means working on each of the additional points (shown in the diagrams on pages 22–23) for ten seconds each. Start your work on the big toe, then work sideways out to the edge of the foot; then move down, towards the heel, to the next line of pressure points and along them, and so on, until all are treated.

Give each sole about five minutes pressure. The right amount of pressure is that which will make you aware of any potential soreness in the points, which indicates congestion in the associated glands and organs, so start gently and then go deeper to find any soreness. Then concentrate especially on the sorest points. If you find that your fingers are not strong enough, use your thumbs or knuckles instead. You may find that a toothbrush handle is effective. If your hands are too weak or stiff, or you cannot reach your feet, someone else can do the pressure work for you. Ideally, you should carry out the treatment twice a day, with the zone stimulation taking about ten minutes for both feet. Working on the tongue can be especially beneficial too as, again, all the body's zones are represented on the tongue and you can often effect a quick response by applying pressure to it or biting it.

Sometimes, the treatment involves work on areas other than the feet. With the condition of asthma or headache, pressure is applied with the thumb into the roof of the mouth. All the body's zones are represented on the roof of the mouth. This will be described on the relevant charts.

Drink a glass of pure water after each session, to flush out any toxins. For many ailments, suggestions for improvements to the diet are given on the chart.

You should continue with the treatment until you get relief from your problem; this will be indicated by soreness disappearing from the zone points treated. This may take a day, a week, a month or longer, depending on the seriousness of the condition, the amount of time you devote to the treatment, and the levels of congestion in the pressure points. With more persistent and chronic conditions, continue as necessary to obtain long-term relief. It is important to emphasize that the treatment is to be used in conjunction with any medical treatment or medication you are receiving, and should not be seen as a substitute. If your condition persists or gets worse, you should consult your medical doctor.

THE THREE-POINT SYSTEM

The three-point system is applied to the ten-minute daily routine, the one-minute pick-me-up and should also be followed when treating any of the ailments listed in the A to Z section.

The procedure is as follows:

> 1. **Tune in to the healing color.**
> 2. **Repeat the "positive permanent thinking replacement".**
> 3. **Start to pressurize the Zone Therapy points.**

Your ten-minute daily routine

Everyone's idea of contentment is to have good health. The greatest gifts from the gods are zest, energy, drive and the glow that comes from perfect health.

We must take responsibility for our bodies and our psyches. The psyche will affect the brain, which will tell the physical body what to do. The body you have now is the only one you're getting in this lifetime, so regard it as a precious commodity. Whether you are in good health now, or fighting an illness or ailment, this simple, three-step daily workout using Color Zone Therapy will enable you to maintain maximum Total Health.

The three steps of the ten-minute treatment
If you are to stop the same ailments or physical problems recurring time and time again, you need to alter your mental state. Your brain is a computer and it will instruct the rest of you.

1. The rainbow of white light

White light comes from the clear brilliance of sunlight, which is the supreme ray, and is the main color used for healing and general clearance. White light acts as an antiseptic and cleanser upon the body. White is a carrier and host to every color. Every organ and gland in the body has its own color, so by using white you will be receiving an equal amount of all of the colors. White is a most beneficial color for maintaining health.

2. Pure thoughts and positive thinking

The second step consists of a positive affirmation to repeat to yourself, enabling you to blot out any negative vibrations that may have crept into your mind. Any negativity that is not dealt with will eventually invade your physical body and cause illness. Because the mind influences every cell in the body, it is imperative that it is given something positive to concentrate on, such as an affirmation. This will steer it back on to the right track. The continuous repetition of energy-charged thoughts through words that are linking with the vibration of color can release the mind from its negative programming, if it has become bogged down, and stuck with unfulfilling attitudes. Every word has its own color and will respond to that color when it is spoken. The affirmations have been specifically chosen to harness the color power of that word. Affirmations can rewrite the program that directs all the cells, so that we can move forward into joy, contentment and full health.

3. Zoning in—the body is your temple

The third step is to treat the Zone Therapy points on the feet; to acquire Total Health you must harness your physical body to the treatment, as well as the spirit and mind. Nine zone points have been chosen for this ten-minute treatment. If you stimulate these points on both feet, shown on the diagrams that follow, you will be stimulating the most important healing points for the glands and organs to ensure optimal health. The zone points relate to the thyroid, pituitary, thymus and adrenal glands, and to the liver, spleen, heart and ovaries or prostate. When you practice on these magical points on your body, you will indeed have the world at your fingertips. Don't forget that this part of the ten-minute treatment can be given to you by someone else if you are not able to do it.

Healing color—RAINBOW WHITE

STEP 1:

Find a comfortable resting place for yourself. Close your eyes and relax. Let all your muscles go, while you concentrate on your breath as it goes in and out slowly.

Imagine that the top of your head is opening, and that a beautiful beam of white light is pouring down into you. This white light will be filling up your body with healing energy. Eventually, after two minutes—not more than this—imagine the pores of your skin opening, so that the light can filter through. As it escapes from your body, this light turns into a soft, pale mist that gently wraps itself around you, forming a cocoon of safety and healing.

STEP 2: POSITIVE AFFIRMATION

Underlying Negative Mental and Emotional Attitude Eliminate:
I feel like a failure.
People don't like me.
People won't accept me the way I am.
I'm a loser.

While in this meditative state of the rainbow white light of energy healing, start to repeat to yourself for those two minutes:

Permanent Positive Thinking Replacement Repeat:
I love life.
Life is a joy, and filled with love.
I love myself and others love me.
Every day, and in every way, I am becoming stronger and stronger.

STEP 3: ZONE THERAPY STIMULATION

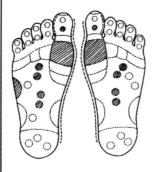

With your eyes open, you are now ready to perform the treatment on both your feet, incorporating the nine healing points.

Start with the points for the pituitary, which is the healing gland; for good health, it should always be in perfect condition. Next, work on the thyroid and parathyroid glands, which are almost as important. Then go on to treat the points for the thymus and adrenal glands, and for the nervous system. Finally, check out the points for the liver and kidneys, and give them treatment if they feel sensitive.

Continue to work on these, even if they seem painful at first. Persevere and, as your general health improves, it will become a daily pleasure to give yourself this treatment. As you work on the nine points, carry on with Steps 1 and 2, so that for the last six minutes of the treatment all three steps will be working in harmony.

Your one-minute pick-me-up

This a quick routine, for times when you find your energy flagging. Again, there are three steps, which you can work on at the same time.

Healing color—BRIGHT RED

STEP 1:

Use the color red, just for one minute.

STEP 2: POSITIVE AFFIRMATION

Realize that feelings of exhaustion are nature's way of saying "I need a break". So the negative response is that you have not paced yourself adequately; there is a deficit in the expansion/contraction rhythm within your system.

Underlying Negative Mental and Emotional Attitude
Eliminate:
Losing trust in all things that are natural.

Permanent Positive Thinking Replacement
Repeat:
I trust the process of life.
Every day, and in every way, I pulsate with the rhythm of
life.

STEP 3: ZONE THERAPY STIMULATION

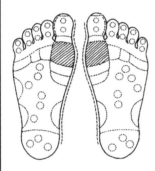

If you can work on your feet, concentrate on the points for the thyroid glands on both feet, under the
big toe.

If this isn't possible, you can
work on the corresponding points
on your ears instead. All the zones
of the body are represented in the
ears. Take the outside rim of one
ear and, starting at the top, apply
strong pressure with your thumb and first finger. Work
down slowly and firmly to the lobe of the ear

HOW TO MEDITATE WITH COLOR

Throughout this book, we have been describing the conscious
and unconscious mind, and how vital it is to work with both
of these for health and wellbeing. So far, we have been dealing with remedies; meditation brings you in touch with your
original source. There is a universal law, which has its own
intelligence, and to which we are all subject; but we have to
live in a society with human-made rules, so we can be led
away from the universal law. The way to get back to the original life force is by meditation. It doesn't matter what religion
or beliefs you hold—none of us can escape the law of nature.

COLOR MEDITATION

Wear loose clothing. Avoid all sources of disturbance. Sit, or lie with your knees drawn up and your feet flat on the floor or bed; close your eyes and let your mind wander for a few minutes. Let a sense of peace and tranquillity fill your entire being. Breathe in and out quietly, and in a completely relaxed way.

Slowly begin to imagine and see with your mind's eye, beautiful colors. See them swirling around within you, for this is your slow introduction to the power within you, as you begin to open your inner universe. Imagine that the top of your head is opening; and beaming down into it is a shimmering ray of a colored light of heavenly dimensions. The color you choose may be, for instance, blue, red or yellow, depending on what condition afflicts you. If you are not working with a particular ailment, you can either choose the white light or whichever color you wish.

As the color reaches your head, it sends out a shower of stars that cascade around you and pour into your body. As it enters you, a glowing feeling of warmth and softness engulfs you. You are full of this beautiful color. It filters down your spine and into your feet. Every part of you is filled with light.

When your body is full, become conscious of your eyes, and see them filling up with the beautiful color. Your eyes become loose, and appear to be floating and bobbing around in their sockets, filled with this colored, healing liquid.

Allow the light to move upwards towards your brain. Let the colored light penetrate deeply, cleansing dark, unwanted spots away as it filters through. The mind is becoming quiet and settling down. Your body will now be filled with this healing colored light. You begin to feel the pores of your body opening and your skin letting the color filter through. It feels like a soft mist that gently touches your face and swirls around your body. It caresses you, cocooning and protecting you in a lovely colored vapor.

If you are working with a particular health condition, repeat the positive thinking affirmations given on the charts of ailments. Dwell upon your feet, your hands, and your face and ears. Focus on the Zone Therapy techniques.

As you come out of your meditative state, feel that the top of your head is closing; this helps you to regulate the power flowing in. Take a few deep breaths in and out, and finally breathe in to the count of four, hold your breath for a count of sixteen, then release and breathe out to a count of eight. Do this exercise twice. These last two breaths bring the oxygen to the brain so that you can be safely earthed again. Then rub both hands together very quickly until you feel them tingling.

This color meditation opens up your mind, as the power within begins to work. It also prepares you for healing. A little time spent meditating brings about peace and deep relaxation, which opens up your physical body to receive help.

Tuning into this, through meditation, will put you in touch with your true self, and bring you the contentment you seek.

If possible, try to find some time each day to meditate. The best time to meditate is usually in the morning before you start your day's activities, or in the evening. You will soon feel the benefits, for you are contacting on a daily basis your mental and emotional bodies. It is a wonderful way of connecting you to inspirational energies, which assist the healing process. You also reach parts of your person you never knew existed and a new way of tapping into directions for your life becomes clear. You begin to channel cosmic energy into your life. You are automatically creating change and that can only enhance your life, and give you access to clear, positive action. Meditation brings you in touch with realms of yourself that you have always known were within you; it brings you closer to your real self. It allows you to become whole again.

As this process develops, you will feel the cumulative effect upon your physical body, for every gland and organ becomes revitalized. Disease is caused by deviation from the universal laws of cause and effect. Rectify this, and you can eliminate disease. If you care for your body and give it consideration it will serve you well. You will also develop the power to create harmonious thought currents, and that will help you along the pathway to wisdom.

A TO Z OF COMMON AILMENTS

There now follows an A to Z listing of common ailments with specific advice for each complaint from which you may be suffering.

AT the physical level, alcohol damages the liver, kidneys, nervous system and brain cells, and these are serious effects. But it is also important to address the underlying emotional issues—the reasons for drinking in the first place, such as the potential of alcohol in enabling you to blot out unbearable "original pain" from past experiences. You should proceed with Color Zone Therapy consistently, for as long as it takes, applying yourself with discipline, vigor and determination—engendering the belief that you really can build a new, alcohol-free life for yourself.

Underlying Negative Mental and Emotional Attitude Eliminate:

There is no structure to my life.
LIFE always lets me down.
What I am is not good enough.
I prefer to live in a different realm.
NOBODY LOVES ME.

Positive Permanent Thinking Replacement
Visualize INDIGO and repeat:

Nobody can tell me what to do.
I am now capable of structuring and creating my divine world of LOVE and ACCEPTANCE.
I LOVE ME.

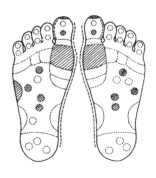

Zone Treatment

The most important glands and organs to treat are the liver and kidneys, the gall bladder and spleen, the adrenal and thymus glands, the thyroids, pituitary gland and brain. You should also work to remove toxins from all the glands and organs in the body to ensure that you can function at 100 percent.

ALLERGIES

Healing Color: YELLOW

ALLERGIES can be difficult to eliminate. If you have an allergy it means that your glandular and organic systems are not functioning properly, and that certain glands or organs have become intolerant of particular substances. Use Zone Therapy to bring every gland and organ up to 100 percent performance and then, if necessary, you can start eliminating specific foods from your diet if you believe the cause lies there.

Underlying Negative Mental and Emotional Attitude
Eliminate:
Suspicious of trusting.
Rejecting life on all levels.
Enraged at the world and its ways.
"Allergic to parents" beliefs.

Positive Permanent Thinking Replacement
Visualize YELLOW and repeat:
I do not have to take on everybody else's problems.
I can see all that is good in the universe and allow myself to reject that which is not.

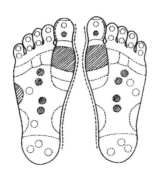

Zone Treatment
The main organs and glands to work on are the pituitary and thyroid glands, the kidneys, liver, adrenals, thymus and nervous system. Concentrate particularly on eliminating any soreness.

ALZHEIMER'S DISEASE

Healing Color: PURPLE

THIS complaint starts with a gradual loss of memory. If caught in its early stages, Zone Therapy can help to slow down its progress by increasing circulation to the brain. It cannot, however, repair brain cells once gone. In the disease's later stages, a relative or friend will need to do the treatment for the sufferer.

Underlying Negative Mental and Emotional Attitude Eliminate:
The belief that I need to control but I cannot.
I cannot face life so I would rather not be here.
As I can't have my own way, I choose to be
SPACED OUT.

Positive Permanent Thinking Replacement Visualize PURPLE *and repeat:*
It is safe for me to be here.
I am in the perfect place at the right time.

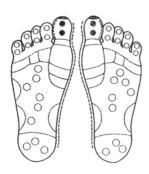

Zone Treatment
The main glands and organs to treat are the brain, the pineal gland and the pituitary gland. It is also important to do a general tone up of all the glands and organs. It may be easier to work on the hands rather than the feet in this instance.

ANAL BLEEDING

Healing Color: BLUE

ANAL bleeding is usually caused by a malfunction in the kidney, bladder or prostate area. It usually responds very quickly to treatment.

Underlying Negative Mental and Emotional Attitude
This condition represents getting everything back to front.
Eliminate:
Giving up too much on life.
Trying too hard.

Positive Permanent Thinking Replacement
Visualize BLUE *and repeat:*
I can let go of trying to be perfect.
Everything is happening in accordance with the
DIVINE PLAN.

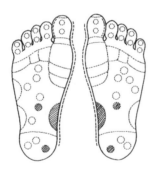

Zone Treatment
Work on the kidneys, the bladder and (for men) the prostate gland. Concentrate especially on the areas where you feel soreness. Give yourself at least five ten-minute treatments a day. Be determined!

ANEMIA

ANEMIA is usually caused by a lack of iron in the blood and in storage in the spleen. If not attended to the condition can turn to pernicious anemia, which is very serious. If your condition is extreme you should see your doctor immediately. Anemia affects more women than men, because women require more iron. Liver and lettuce are rich in iron, and daily sources of vitamin C will help in its absorption.

Underlying Negative Mental and Emotional Attitude
The blood is the body's life force. Blood deficiencies represent loss of power somewhere in your life.
Eliminate:
Feeling inferior.
Losing the will to live.

Positive Permanent Thinking Replacement
Visualize RED ***and repeat:***
I take back all that belongs to me with strength and vigor.
I will seize the day for myself always.

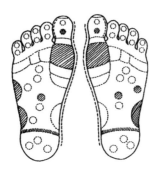

Zone Treatment
Work especially on the areas for the spleen. Concentrate on really rotating your thumb on these areas, working with determination. The spleen has a great effect on the intestines so you should also work on the ascending, descending and sigmoid colon, liver, adrenals, pituitary and thyroid glands. Working on all the glands and organs will give you an extra boost on the road to recovery.

ANGINA

Healing Color: GREEN

THE treatment for this condition can be applied very simply and will help to relieve the pain of an attack. It works by moving all congestion from the areas that affect the heart and by helping to calm your nervous system. You must consult your doctor if you have this condition.

Underlying Negative Mental and Emotional Attitude
Angina represents a warning to let go of unnecessary chores in your life. Think of it as reassessment time.
Eliminate:
Not good at pacing myself.
A tired heart.

Positive Permanent Thinking Replacement
Visualize GREEN ***and repeat:***
There is a time and place for everything.
I can now go with the **flow** of life with **ease**.

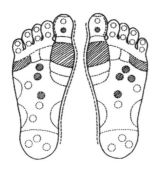

Zone Treatment
Work on the heart and lungs, the nervous system, the adrenal glands, the thymus gland, the thyroid and pituitary glands. You may find it more convenient to work on the hands for this condition.

ARTHRITIS Healing Color: ORANGE

ARTHRITIS is caused by too much acidity building up in the body. The kidneys can therefore become very congested. The first thing to do with arthritis is to change your diet—cut out all acidity—that is, uric acid (red meat), lactic acid (milk) and citric acid (citrus fruit). To purify your system, put a tablespoon each of black molasses, cider vinegar and honey into a cup, add hot water, stir and drink. Do this at least twice a day.

Exercise as much as you can and keep your joints moving.

Underlying Negative Mental and Emotional Attitude
The emotional aspect of this problem usually stems from early sibling rivalry—jealousies. Your experience of life would be not getting your share.

Eliminate:
Not accepted.
Resentment.
It was not fair.
Forced to do things against one's will.

Positive Permanent Thinking Replacement
Visualize ORANGE *and repeat:*
I can let go of the blame and forgive the past.
I have **joy** and **acceptance** now.

Zone Treatment

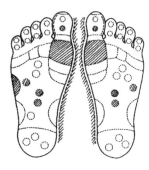

Work mainly on the kidneys and the thyroid gland. The kidneys eliminate acidity from the body and the thyroid helps to bring the nervous system under control, thus helping the stress-related aspect of the condition. Also treat the liver, gall bladder, adrenal glands, spleen, ileocecal valve, pituitary gland, and all back, shoulder and hip areas.

ASTHMA
Healing Color: ORANGE

ASTHMA is caused by a malfunction of the adrenal glands and the nervous system. As with sinus problems, catarrh and bronchial troubles and hay fever, you may also be troubled by imperfect nasal passages. If this is the case, see a nose and head specialist, and have your nose examined.

Underlying Negative Mental and Emotional Attitude
Asthma can be an unintentional emotional transferral of the mother's anxieties on to the child. As the saying goes—"Heal the mother, Heal the child".
Eliminate:
CONFINED.
Overloaded with responsibilities.
Trying to make things right for others.

Positive Permanent Thinking Replacement
Visualize ORANGE and repeat:
I do not have to give up MYSELF to please others.
I am free to do as I WANT.

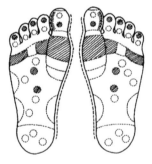

Zone Treatment
Work first on the areas for the adrenal, pituitary and thyroid glands, and the nervous system. The lungs, bronchial and sinus areas will also need attention.

In addition, press firmly into the roof of the mouth with your thumb. Press all over the inside of the top of the mouth for three minutes; then rest for a minute and repeat. Next, take the handle of a dessert spoon or toothbrush, and put pressure on the tongue, beginning as far back as you can without gagging. Apply pressure all over the tongue, right up to the tip, for a three-minute period. Do all this twice a day.

Finally, also bite on the tip of the tongue (which relates to the bronchial tract) every time you remember to.

BACK PROBLEMS

Healing Color: INDIGO

THE back is very susceptible to injury. In your body you have 214 bones connected in different ways to the spine, and any injury to the back affects the sympathetic nervous system, your muscles, organs and glands and, of course, the central nervous system. Toxins will have accumulated on your nerve endings, blocking the electromagnetic force that keeps you alive, so strong Zone Therapy treatment is required.

Underlying Negative Mental and Emotional Attitude

High back and shoulder problems
(the shoulders are the corners of happiness)

Eliminate:
Taking on too much.
Life is a big burden.
Get off my back.
Put upon.

Mid back problems

Eliminate:
Emotional problems and let downs,
usually **relationships**.

Lower back problems

Eliminate:
Insecurity, usually **money** problems.
Poverty may be a state of mind, but it gets you in the back.
No **structure** to life.

Positive Permanent Thinking Replacements

High back and shoulder problems

Visualize INDIGO *and repeat:*
I now have confidence to throw off life's burdens.
I take on board only tender feelings of JOY.

Mid back problems

Visualize INDIGO *and repeat:*
As I love myself unconditionally,
I am now ready to give and receive
LOVE.

Lower back problems

Visualize INDIGO *and repeat:*
I can now make my own rules.
I will not hold myself back in
LIFE.

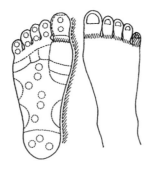

Zone Treatment
Start by working on the sore points from the base of the spine which runs along the ridge of the inside of the foot. Do all that area, then work up all the inside ridge of the foot right up to where the big toe joins the foot—that corresponds to the complete spine, from bottom to top. Massage the entire area until the soreness is eliminated.

For the back of the neck and the shoulders, work across the back top of the foot, where all the toes join the feet, including the big toes. The backs of the little toes are the areas for the shoulder joints so massage these too.

The neck area is where the big toe joins the foot. If you have a neck problem, massage deep into that part.

The outer ankle represents the hip joints, so massage the outside of the ankle for any hip problem.

You must be determined, and you must be very positive. Put the pressure on with your fingers and thumbs; do not be weak about it—be strong, because you have to break down the blockage around your nerve endings as quickly as possible.

BAD breath is often caused by a poor diet, so cut out any junk food, take a good laxative, and eat plenty of fruit and vegetables, all as fresh as possible. Drink at least eight large glasses of water and follow a regular routine of physical exercises every day.

Other culprits could be a malfunctioning pancreas, a faulty liver or kidneys, or colonic trouble.

Underlying Negative Mental and Emotional Attitude
Eliminate:
Rotten thoughts.
Stagnant ideas.
Something from the past still FERMENTING.

Positive Permanent Thinking Replacement
Visualize YELLOW and repeat:
I can start afresh.
I am youth and joy.
I am **reborn**.
I feel a **cleansing** of my **soul**.

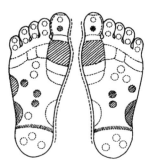

Zone Treatment
The main areas to work on are all related to the digestive system and include the ascending colon, descending colon, sigmoid colon, liver, kidneys, gall bladder, spleen, and adrenal, thyroid and pituitary glands.

BINGING

Healing Color: GREEN

BINGING indicates a deep-seated emotional problem which you will need to address. On a practical level, discipline and control are essential to help you cut out junk foods. Binging causes digestive problems and high levels of toxicity in the body which need to be dealt with.

Underlying Negative Mental and Emotional Attitude
Binging literally fills a gap. It is a substitute for not being able to get your own way.
Eliminate:
Famine in emotional life.
A fear of success.
Needing protection.

Positive Permanent Thinking Replacement
Visualize GREEN ***and repeat:***
It is safe to be me.
I can trust myself at all times.
The Universe loves me just as I am.

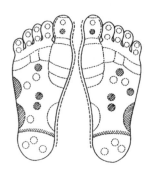

Zone Treatment
The main glands and organs to treat are the liver and kidneys, the spleen and colons, and the adrenal, thymus and pituitary glands.

BLOOD PRESSURE

HIGH BLOOD PRESSURE	Healing Color: BLUE
LOW BLOOD PRESSURE	Healing Color: RED

BLOOD pressure can be a problem especially in later years, because the walls of the blood vessels become smaller. The danger is that the pressure against the walls of the blood vessels greatly increases, which can cause a blood vessel to break. When this happens, real trouble begins, because a clot can be formed and lodge in the small capillaries of the brain, leading to paralysis, or in the heart area, causing angina.

Blood pressure is the result of the balance created by the glands and organs that should supply the correct amount of adrenalin and hormones for the circulation to create proper chemical stability. There are other factors, too—if elimination is poor, congestion will build up and abnormal amounts of calcium, for instance, will stick to the walls of the arteries. The result will be abnormal elasticity. The effort required by the heart is therefore increased.

People suffering from high blood pressure should try not to allow themselves to be put under nervous stress. You need peace of mind. Do not get into a worked-up state emotionally because it can cause the walls of the blood vessels to contract. So for people with high blood pressure, the message is keep calm, and walk away from it, whatever the cause. By removing tension from your life, following the recommendations here and also toning up your entire glandular system, you will be able to achieve very good results with this problem.

Underlying Negative Mental and Emotional Attitude

High blood pressure

Eliminate:
Suppressed anger over a **long period of time**.

Low blood pressure

Eliminate:
Defeatism.
What's the use, I've given up.
Unhappiness.

Positive Permanent Thinking Replacement

High blood pressure
Visualize BLUE *and repeat:*
Now is the time to fully express my **power** and **strength**.

Low blood pressure
Visualize RED *and repeat:*
I love me as I am.
I am **perfect** just as I am.

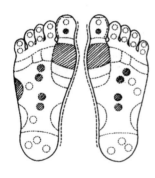

Zone Treatment
The treatment will bring your blood pressure back to a normal healthy level from either a high or a low state. Work on your liver, kidneys, thyroid, adrenal, pituitary and thymus glands and, especially, your nervous system.

BREAST CANCER

Healing Color: INDIGO

IN addition to the general treatment mentioned under the heading "Cancer" on pages 75–76, you can also follow this more specific routine. If you are receiving chemotherapy, it is especially important to visualize the healing color during the sessions. Remember that Color Zone Therapy is there to assist and not to replace your normal treatment.

Underlying Negative Mental and Emotional Attitude
Eliminate:
FRUSTRATION.
Not being acknowledged in any areas in my life.
A belief that I can only be loved for what I do,
and not for who I am.
Extreme irritation.
I must keep working.

Positive Permanent Thinking Replacement
Visualize INDIGO and repeat:
I can see the green fields of home.
This place is mine, and the Universe knows it.
It is just fine to ease myself into
NEEDED REST.

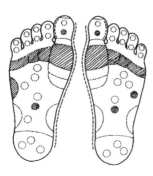

Zone Treatment
Work primarily on the points for the lungs, chest and bronchial areas. It is also very important to have every gland or organ functioning at 100 percent capacity to enable you to fight the disease and create new, healthy cells as quickly as possible. Focus on the pituitary and thyroid glands, and on the liver, kidneys and spleen.

PROBLEMS such as breast lumps are naturally very worrying; although they are very often non-active, you should always consult your medical doctor at the same time as using Color Zone Therapy.

Underlying Negative Mental and Emotional Attitude
The female breast represents nurturing, tenderness and caring, and the flowing milk of kindness.
Eliminate:
Lack of nurturing for oneself.
A belief that it's better to be a man.

Positive Permanent Thinking Replacement
Visualize INDIGO *and repeat:*
I glorify in my femininity, softness and roundness.
I am a powerful woman.

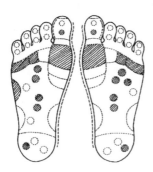

Zone Treatment
The treatment points are those for the lungs, chest and nervous systems, the heart, pituitary and thyroid glands, thymus gland, adrenal glands, ovaries, liver and kidneys. Work until soreness has been eliminated.

BRONCHITIS | Healing Color: INDIGO

BRONCHITIS is a condition which affects the bronchial tract in the chest area. Color Zone Therapy helps by easing the congestion in the lungs and chest. Inhaling steam is also a great help—put a few drops of vapor rub into a bowl or basin of very hot water. Place a towel over your head and inhale the steam. Do this three or four times a week.

Underlying Negative Mental and Emotional Attitude
The bronchial tubes are passageways for the air to the lungs.
They represent your path in life.
Inflammation causes a blockage along the pathways.
Eliminate:
Congestion on the road to success.
Caged.
Imprisoned.

Positive Permanent Thinking Replacement
Visualize INDIGO and repeat:
I can travel through life and meet all that
comes with **hope** and **excitement**.

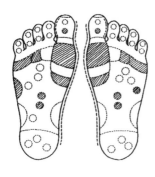

Zone Treatment
Work primarily on the lung and all chest areas. To improve your general levels of health, also work on the thyroid, pituitary and adrenal glands, as well as the liver, kidneys, spleen and pancreas. The tip of the tongue relates straight down to the bronchial tract so biting on it gently several times a day can also help.

BRUISES

BRUISING is usually nature's reminder that you have been careless! So the first thing is to pay more attention to your actions—change carelessness into quick perception. When you go into a room look around, then close your eyes and remember straight away what you have seen. Practice this art until you have instant recall. You have to be more careful.

Underlying Negative Mental and Emotional Attitude
Misplaced judgements are a strong reminder that there is a need to think again.
Eliminate:
Self-neglect and punishment.
A belief of not being good enough.
Not paying attention to yourself.

Positive Permanent Thinking Replacement
Visualize INDIGO ***and repeat:***
I rejoice in the constant care I give myself.
I can consider myself a part of life's
richness.

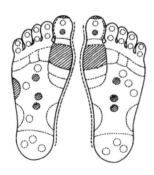

Zone Treatment
It is important to bring your circulation back to 100 percent by working on all the glands and organs. Concentrate especially on the brain, the pituitary, thyroid and adrenal glands, the nervous system, liver and kidneys.

CANCER	Healing Color: GREEN
	(but see caution below)

THIS technique may aid other treatments you are using to deal with cancer. It will not disrupt your medical treatment; you can help your condition by bringing every gland and organ, even those not affected, up to strength. This should make you feel fit enough to take your radiotherapy and chemotherapy. Remember that chemotherapy kills off cells; by toning up your glandular and organic systems, you help your body to create new cells as quickly as possible. Don't just think about it, do it. You have to be as strong as you can possibly manage, to beat your condition.

The Healing Color Treatment: A Word of Caution

You need to meditate every day, using the color green. How to do this is explained in Chapter 4 of this book. But do use the green color sparingly on anything that is malignant; it is best to work with visualizing it for only ten minutes a day. You can use it for one session of ten minutes or break the time up into several sessions. Green can help restore stability to anything malignant, which results from cells that have accelerated out of control. But if overused, it can have a soporific effect on the healthy cells.

Underlying Negative Mental and Emotional Attitude
Eliminate:
Too much acceptance.
Coping—helplessness.
Self-denial. Life is on hold.
The body will move forward and grow,
even if it has to produce **a cancer**.

Positive Permanent Thinking Replacement
Visualize GREEN and repeat:
I will not deny myself the experience and right to a
full and active life.

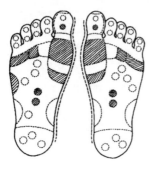

Zone Treatment

Work over all the points on the feet, especially on the lungs, chest, thyroid and pituitary glands, liver, kidneys, pancreas and adrenal glands. Bring them all up to 100 percent. Spend at least ten minutes on each foot, making it a twenty-minute treatment. Make yourself do it or get someone else to do it for you. You could also apply pressure over your tongue with a dessertspoon handle, from the tip of your tongue to as far back as possible without gagging.

Color Treatment for Tumors

For anyone who has a tumor within the body, try using this color treatment:

CANCEROUS TUMORS

Healing Color: INDIGO

THE intention of this simple process is to help you focus on dispersing tumors of any kind. Just close your eyes, as in the meditation process described in Chapter 3, and imagine flowing through your bloodstream little indigo-colored warriors, filtering through the growth. Your indigo ARMY can be anything you like. It can be a band of ravenous fish swallowing all in its way or tiny soldiers armed with spears which break up blockages. After your mine sweepers have detected and blown the tumors out of existence, you can follow it with a visualized green wash flowing through the body, flushing and clearing the debris out.

You need a positive attitude—total faith, being committed to success.

CATARACTS

THERE is no known way to stop a cataract once it is full blown. However, you can help strengthen other parts of your eyes, by working on all eye points to stimulate muscles and the optic nerve. Eventually you will have to have the cataracts removed, but you will have done an excellent job on your eyes that will stand you in good stead afterwards.

Eliminate whole milk products from your diet.

Underlying Negative Mental and Emotional Attitude Eliminate:
Not wanting to look at the future.
Pessimistic.

Positive Permanent Thinking Replacement Visualize INDIGO *and repeat:*
I can see clearly now.
I have faith to look ahead with
anticipation and joy.
My future is **rosy.**

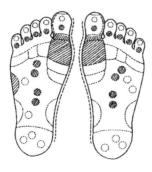

Zone Treatment
Give yourself treatment to the top joints on all your toes. The top joints of the toes relate to all the zones. See that you eliminate all tender spots in those areas.

Work all over the kidneys and at the base of all the toes, then go on to the liver, adrenal and thymus glands, nervous system, thyroid and pituitary glands.

CATARRH

FIRST of all, you may need to check with your doctor that you have no obstructions in your nose.

Pay attention to breathing properly—always breathe in and out through your nose. This is vital for filtering out any dust and dirt which could otherwise cause catarrh.

To get rid of catarrh, you must clean out your whole system. You must look to your diet—no more junk food. Cut out all the full milk products (try skimmed or soy milk instead), chocolates, sweets and biscuits as these are all mucus producing. You need to eat lots of fresh salads, good green vegetables and tons of fresh fruit. You need eight large glasses of mineral water every day.

Underlying Negative Mental and Emotional Attitude
Eliminate:
Sticky thinking.
Clinging on to nothing.
Making a **molehill** into a **mountain**.

Positive Permanent Thinking Replacement
Visualize ORANGE *and repeat:*
I trust the path I have chosen.
Everything is evolving exactly to plan.
Look out world, here I come.
I am a winner.

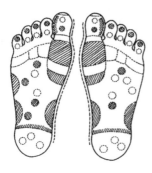

Zone Treatment
Work all over your sinus points. Then, to aid elimination of toxins and to clean up your whole system, focus on the pituitary, thyroid and thymus glands, and pancreas. Finally, work on your liver, kidneys, ileocecal valve, bladder, gall bladder and colons.

CELLULITE

CELLULITE occurs when your body cannot process waste properly. Detoxification is necessary, so dietary changes and increasing your intake of drinking water may be required. Drink eight glasses of pure water every day. Eat plenty of fruit and vegetables. Embark on a full program of exercise. Include plenty of leg and thigh exercise, such as cycling or walking uphill.

If the total Color Zone program and the above recommendations are followed persistently, you can expect excellent results.

Underlying Negative Mental and Emotional Attitude
Eliminate:
Stored-up failure.
Banked-up rubbish in the psyche.
Hidden skeletons in the closet.
Fear of being found out.

Positive Permanent Thinking Replacement
Visualize YELLOW *and repeat:*
My mistakes are my greatest teacher,
I dissolve them all with
LOVE and GRATITUDE.

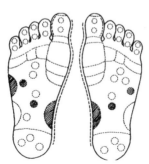

Zone Treatment
To help your body eliminate accumulated poisons and to purify your whole system you need to work on the areas shown for the liver, kidneys, spleen, bladder, gall bladder and lymphatic system.

CHOLESTEROL Healing Color: YELLOW

DIET is the most important factor in the level of blood cholesterol, which mainly affects the heart and circulation, though other glands and organs play a part too.

The main sources of cholesterol are fatty foods such as butter and margarine, chocolates, fatty meat and anything fried. Remove these from your diet. However, excessive protein is also a factor. Reduce your intake; steamed fish or breast of chicken are acceptable. Ensure that 90 percent of your diet consists of fresh vegetables and fruit. Drink eight glasses of pure water daily.

If you suffer from very high cholesterol, consult your doctor.

Underlying Negative Mental and Emotional Attitude
Eliminate:
Lack of enthusiasm.
Always being disappointed.
Fear of daring.
Nothing works out right for
me.

Positive Permanent Thinking Replacement
Visualize YELLOW *and repeat:*
All doors and channels are wide open for me.
It's my turn now.
I enter, and move along with **hope** and **happiness**.

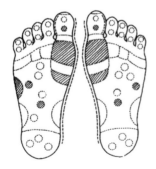

Zone Treatment
Work especially on the areas shown for the heart and chest. Also treat the areas for the thyroid and pituitary glands to help stimulate your whole system. Treat your body's filters—the organ areas for the liver, kidneys, spleen, pancreas and gall bladder.

CIRCULATION   Healing Color: YELLOW

MANY people suffer from poor circulation; in the winter chilblains are the result, and even in the summertime hands and feet can be consistently cold. As always, consult your doctor—you may need to increase your intake of iron.

Your diet needs to include good protein, backed up with lots of fresh fruit and green vegetables. Exercise is vitally important. If you can only manage a good brisk walk, that will help .

Underlying Negative Mental and Emotional Attitude
Eliminate:
Lack of joy in my life.
Nothing special ever happens to me.
I have nowhere to go.
Uninvited.

Positive Permanent Thinking Replacement
Visualize YELLOW and repeat:
I can flow freely to the movement of my blood **singing**.
The world is my oyster.

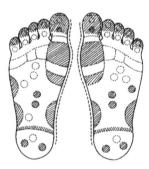

Zone Treatment
To improve your circulation you must work well on your liver, kidneys, adrenal glands, pancreas, spleen, all the thyroids, pituitary, prostate or ovaries, bladder, and all colons. Apply pressure to the top joints of each toe to stimulate circulation through all the zones.

Use a soft wire brush to stroke up your arms over the back of the hands, and also up your legs from the top of your feet. Do this for a few minutes morning and night. Always stroke upwards. Massage the ears all over between fingers and thumb for a few moments each day (each gland and organ has a nerve ending in the ear). This treatment will also improve your entire nervous system.

COLIC

COLIC is mainly caused by impurities in food or water. If you suspect you have colic, you should consult your medical doctor. But you can meanwhile pursue Color Zone Therapy treatment with advantage.

The state of the colon is of primary importance. Diet is crucial too. Eliminate junk foods completely from your diet. Eat plenty of vegetables, salads and soft fruits, all as fresh as possible. Drink eight glasses of pure water a day. It should not be chilled; if you can manage to drink warm water, this is better still.

Underlying Negative Mental and Emotional Attitude
Eliminate:
Agitation.
Holding down extreme hurt.
Always doing the dirty work.
Being the MARTYR.

Positive Permanent Thinking Replacement
Visualize BLUE *and repeat:*
I give myself permission to
LAUGH.

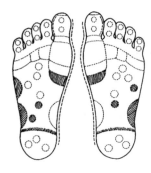

Zone Treatment
Work on all the colon areas, as well as the other organs of digestion, the liver, kidneys, spleen, pancreas and ileocecal valve. Also treat the areas for all the glands to bring you back to full health.

If you are treating a baby for colic, use the flat of your hand and work all over the feet except for the toes.

AS with colic, the most important organ to treat is of course the colon. To help purification, drink eight large glasses of pure water each day and take a tablespoonful of black molasses at least twice a day, in a cup of hot water.

Underlying Negative Mental and Emotional Attitude Eliminate:
Emotional inflammation.
Sick with putting up with dishonesty.
Everyone expects too much from me.
Workaholic.

Positive Permanent Thinking Replacement Visualize BLUE *and repeat:*
I am perfect just as I am.
I can now take a smooth passage
through life.
I am PEACE.

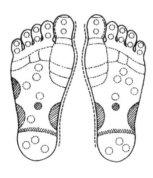

Zone Treatment
Treat all the areas pertaining to the colon—sigmoid, ascending and descending. Also work on the areas for the liver, kidneys and bladder.

COMMON COLD

ISN'T it amazing that, after all this time, there is still no cure for the common cold—with the total inconvenience and devastation it causes? Fortunes are spent every day on remedies, to no avail; that little virus keeps right on to the end of the road.

What is the best cure for a cold? The answer is quite simple: PREVENTION. If you keep every gland and organ up to scratch, and take high doses of vitamin C, you will be well on the road to keeping colds at bay. Also, drink eight large, very hot cups of good water every day—as hot as you can manage to drink comfortably.

If you do succumb, get into a really warm bed, well enough wrapped up to induce a good sweat. If you follow this routine, a couple of days will see you over the difficulty.

Underlying Negative Mental and Emotional Attitude
Eliminate:
Being stretched in too many directions at once.
Scattered thoughts.
A **breakdown** in the **running order**.

Positive Permanent Thinking Replacement
Visualize GREEN *and repeat:*
I can focus on what is best for me in a calm and
relaxed manner.
There is time to fit in all I need to do.

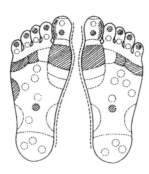

Zone Treatment
Work upon the lungs, the chest and all sinus points. Pay particular attention to the lungs and sinuses, for they will be tender and sore to touch. Work upon the pituitary and thyroid glands to stimulate your immune system. Give the liver and kidneys a good working over to help purify your system.

TO exercise your eyes, fill the wash-hand basin with clean cold water and, with your eyes open, take a deep breath and put your face in the water for a few seconds at a time. Keeping your eyes open, move them around and about. This will help eye complaints enormously.

Rest your eyes, and do not watch television or go to the cinema until your condition has cleared.

Underlying Negative Mental and Emotional Attitude
Eliminate:
Sore at life.
Everything is a strain.
Not wanting to look at the situation.

Positive Permanent Thinking Replacement
Visualize INDIGO *and repeat:*
My life is looking good.
I am looking good.
I see only beauty in my life and in
myself.

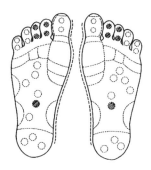

Zone Treatment
Work over the eye points at the base of the toes, also the kidneys as these are closely associated with the eyes. Hold the pressure for as long as you can. If you can manage it for a minute you are doing well.

CONSTIPATION   Healing Color: YELLOW

THE first thing to do is look hard at your diet. Stop eating rubbish. Cut out white bread and go for wholemeal instead. You must eat food that contains a high fibre content—also plenty of green vegetables and lots of fresh fruit and stewed prunes. Use pure virgin oil in cooking and dressings; this will help to lubricate the system. Drink at least eight glasses of water daily.

You must exercise—if possible go for a good walk each day, and really take long strides. Hold your stomach in and pull it up while you are walking. Get used to pulling your stomach in and up at all times, even when watching television. If you are fit enough, do plenty of sit-ups.

Underlying Negative Mental and Emotional Attitude
Eliminate:
Hanging on to the past.
Refusing to budge.
There is never enough,
I must hang on **to what I have got**.

Positive Permanent Thinking Replacement
Visualize YELLOW and repeat:
I can let go of all that does not serve me.
I believe in the divine abundance
which allows new ideas to enter my body.

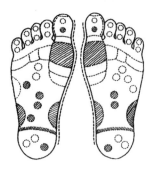

Zone Treatment
Work on all the colon points, the ileo-cecal valve, the kidneys, the bladder and prostate points, the gall bladder, the thyroid and pituitary glands, and the adrenal glands.

With a dessertspoon handle give firm pressure all over the tongue for a few minutes at least twice a day.

CYSTITIS

CYSTITIS is an upsetting complaint of the urinary system. It helps to drink as much hot water as you can.

Underlying Negative Mental and Emotional Attitude
Eliminate:
I am fed up with life.
I feel weakened by circumstances.

Positive Permanent Thinking Replacement
Visualize YELLOW *and repeat:*
I am steadfast and true
now that I feel safe and
STRONG TO HOLD MY OWN GROUND.

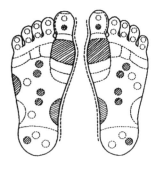

Zone Treatment
Work must be done on your bladder, the kidneys, ovary regions, liver, adrenals, thymus and nervous system. You must work out all soreness, especially in the bladder and kidney areas, until those areas are no longer tender to the touch.

Also work upon the thyroid and pituitary glands to stimulate circulation and raise your spirits.

Give yourself two treatments a day lasting fifteen minutes each time.

Put pressure on the tongue using the handle of a large spoon. Pay particular attention to the centre of the tongue. Apply pressure for thirty seconds, rest for ten seconds, then repeat. Do this four times at each treatment.

DANDRUFF
Healing Color: PURPLE

THIS is mostly caused by pollution in the atmosphere, combined with sweat from the scalp. This creates a scale which does fasten on to the scalp. Be sure to wash your hair regularly, and use a good stiff brush daily on the scalp to loosen and remove all the dust and scaling.

Every evening you should give your scalp a good massaging with your hands or, better still, get someone else to do it for you. Rub glycerine and olive oil in equal amounts into the scalp.

You also need lots of green vegetables and plenty of fresh fruit and good clean water—eight glasses a day.

Underlying Negative Mental and Emotional Attitude
Eliminate:
Unsolved worries.
Anxious.
Not being recognized.
Suppressed talent and intelligence.

Positive Permanent Thinking Replacement
Visualize PURPLE and repeat:
My ideas are clear and bright.
It is a delight to receive them.

Zone Treatment
To stimulate your scalp, you should buffer your finger nails together as hard as possible for fifteen minutes a day. Not all in one go—a few minutes here and there, adding up to fifteen minutes a day. The nerve endings to your scalp are under your nails and need stimulating. If you work in this way, the results will amaze you.

DEAFNESS — Healing Color: YELLOW

EAR problems can often be helped successfully. If you are determined enough, you can mostly be successful with this treatment. You must be prepared to work consistently until you achieve results.

Underlying Negative Mental and Emotional Attitude Eliminate:
The ears will reject and shut out cruel blasts and sounds.
I do not wish to hear.
Please do not disturb me.

Positive Permanent Thinking Replacement
Visualize YELLOW *and repeat:*
I hear only the sounds that are music to my ears.
Music that soothes my soul.

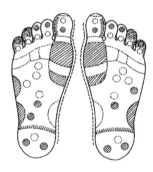

Zone Treatment
The third and fourth toes relating to the ears need attention. Apply pressure with your fingers and thumbs; if you cannot get enough pressure, use the handle of a toothbrush. Press all over the top joints of those toes, removing all the tenderness that exists in those areas, and also put pressure on the sides of the toes.

Use the back of an aluminum comb over the tips of the feet, and hold for a few seconds.

Put pressure over the tongue, particularly over the afflicted parts—that is, the side that has the ear trouble.

You should also work all over the sinus points and the areas of the liver, kidneys, pituitary, thyroid, pancreas, spleen, ileocecal valve, colons, and prostate or ovaries.

Also massage your ear lobes very well. Any tenderness must be worked out.

DEPRESSION Healing Color: YELLOW

SORT out first of all what is making you depressed and face up to it, then be very determined in a fair way to try and alter the situation.

You have to whip up some enthusiasm and get cracking. You can get over this if you put your mind to it.

Underlying Negative Mental and Emotional Attitude Eliminate:
Life is on hold, called to a halt.
Repressed anger and underneath that extreme grief.
No movement.
Static.
Devoid of color.

Positive Permanent Thinking Replacement
Visualize YELLOW *and repeat:*
I can feel joy bubbling up within me.
All things are bright and beautiful.
It is safe for **me** to **move** to the **rhythm** of **life**.

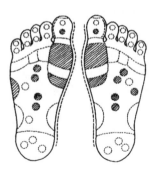

Zone Treatment
Depression affects the whole of your glandular system. Work on the points for the pituitary, thyroids, adrenals, nervous system, pancreas, spleen, liver, kidneys and thymus.

DIABETES

DIABETES is brought on by a malfunction of the pancreas which fails to produce enough insulin. It can sometimes develop in people under the age of thirty, and is treated by insulin injections and diet. It can of course develop at any age if insufficient insulin is being produced. Early symptoms to look for are thirst, blurred vision, tiredness, genital irritation and weight loss.

Zone Therapy can help diabetes but always seek medical advice. If you are already taking insulin, pay heed to the fact that when the pancreas starts to supply insulin into the bloodstream, in addition to the insulin already being taken, procedure must be followed as for insulin shock. Your own physician will recommend an immediate intake of extra sugar for this.

Underlying Negative Mental and Emotional Attitude Eliminate:
Lacks the taste of the sweet life.
No control over events.
Always saying yes to everything.

Positive Permanent Thinking Replacement
Visualize YELLOW *and repeat:*
I now take my power and feel the sweet strength of saying **no**.
I am very good at getting my needs met.

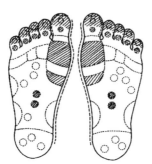

Zone Treatment
Treat the pancreas but remember to work gently. Also treat the pituitary, thyroids, kidneys, adrenals, and all eye and ear areas.

Give pressure over all the top joints of the toes. Then, using the thumb and first finger, massage all over both ears, working out all tender spots.

With the handle of a large spoon, give pressure all over the tongue, in particular the side.

DIARRHEA — Healing Color: INDIGO

DIARRHEA is a sign of malfunction in the digestive system. Eating plenty of ripe bananas can help.

Do stomach exercises; keep pulling your stomach in and up as hard as you can whilst you are walking, standing, sitting or flat out on the floor or bed. You must get some movement; if you are prepared to work at it, you will obtain some results.

Underlying Negative Mental and Emotional Attitude Eliminate:
I just can't hold on to myself.
Life is running away from me.
Fear of death.
Rejection of self.

Positive Permanent Thinking Replacement Visualize INDIGO *and repeat:*
My body works at its own pace,
in its own way.
There is plenty of time to do what
I have to do.

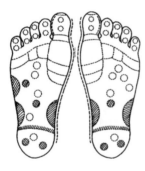

Zone Treatment
Press the sacrum area (the sacrum is the bottom of the back) hard and keep the pressure on for a thirty second period. Then release and rest for a few seconds. Repeat several times a day.

Work on all the colons—the ascending colon, the descending colon, the sigmoid colon.

Then work on the kidneys and bladder, ovaries or prostate, liver and gall bladder.

DIZZINESS   Healing Color: INDIGO

HAVE your eyes and ears checked out with your doctor; also your blood pressure.

Underlying Negative Mental and Emotional Attitude
Eliminate:
Confusion.
Not wanting to face up to responsibilities.
Do not want to be where you are right now.

Positive Permanent Thinking Replacement
Visualize INDIGO *and repeat:*
I am centered and perfectly safe and happy.
I love being in this place right now
this minute.

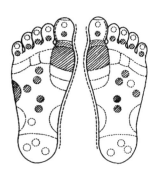

Zone Treatment
The primary treatment is that all ear and eye nerves must be massaged.

Treat the liver, kidneys, spleen, pituitary and neck area; also the thyroids, nervous system, thymus, adrenals and gall bladder.

EAR PROBLEMS

Healing Color: YELLOW

EAR conditions can often be helped and hearing improved with Color Zone Therapy. (See also "Tinnitus" on *p. 153*.)

In addition to the Zone Therapy work below, pressure on the jaw behind the wisdom teeth can be of great benefit to the ears. Place the thumb on the upper jaw at the back of the mouth and apply pressure for a few minutes, or place a little pad of handkerchief or cotton wool behind the wisdom teeth and bite hard on it for a couple of minutes.

Also, with your thumb and first finger, work any tenderness out of the ear lobes and massage the entire ear, back and front.

Underlying Negative Mental and Emotional Attitude
Eliminate:
Irritated at what I hear and all around me.
Not wanting to hear the unpleasant truths.
Discard stubbornness.

Positive Permanent Thinking Replacement
Visualize YELLOW *and repeat:*
I have the ability to create balance
and allow in only what
I want to hear.

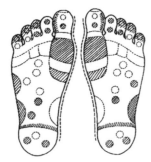

Zone Treatment
Work must be done on the top joints and tips of the third, fourth and little toes, all of which relate to the ears. Also work on the eye reflexes and the sinus areas. Put pressure on to the liver, kidneys, pancreas, pituitary, thyroids, spleen, ileocecal valve, colons and prostate or ovaries.

Using the handle of a large spoon, put on pressure all over the tongue, giving extra attention to the side where deafness is ringing.

EMPHYSEMA Healing Color: INDIGO

PEOPLE who suffer from this chronic congestion of the lungs should immediately give up smoking. Failure to do so can have dramatic consequences.

As a daily exercise, lie down on the bed, place your hands on the stomach and breathe quietly in through the nose; feel the stomach swell, then breathe out through the nose. Become relaxed and calm. All the time, see the color INDIGO. Begin with five to ten minutes and each day add a minute or two, until half an hour is reached.

Underlying Negative Mental and Emotional Attitude
You may feel life has short changed you but there is no reason to continue punishing yourself by becoming short of breath.
Eliminate:
Inferiority complex.
Austere beginnings, not used to kindness.
Deprived of opportunity.

Positive Permanent Thinking Replacement
Visualize INDIGO and repeat:
I am ready to receive unconditional
LOVE from the universe.
I shall breathe fully into my lungs the
sweet air of freedom.
I am in harmony with myself.

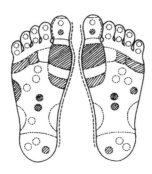

Zone Treatment
Apply pressure over the lungs and chest areas on the feet; massage well into these areas. Then work upon the liver, kidneys and spleen, the pituitary, thyroid, pancreas, adrenals and prostate glands. This will help rid your body of toxins.

FIBROIDS

Healing Color: ORANGE

THIS condition is usually characterized by excessively heavy periods, cramping, and possibly miscarriage; yet the common medical response is all too often "wait till your menopause, and maybe it will disappear'; and the only "treatment" recommended may be hysterectomy. Color Zone Therapy can do a lot better than this.

Underlying Negative Mental and Emotional Attitude Eliminate:
Invasion by others into one's personal life.
Intruded upon.
No respect from others.

Positive Permanent Thinking Replacement Visualize ORANGE *and repeat:*
I welcome all that is good for me with
enthusiasm
and I can reject with ease the rest.
I can now experience life **fully and freely**.

Process: Use the dispersing process for tumors and growths given on page 76, using the color INDIGO.

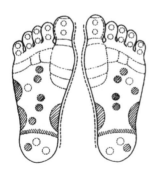

Zone Treatment
Work upon the main organs in the stomach area—all colons, particularly the sigmoid colon, ascending colon and the descending colon—the ovaries, bladder, kidneys, spleen, liver, adrenals and the nervous system and thymus.

Treatment in the ileocecal valve must be done for purification purposes.

FRIGIDITY

FRIGIDITY, lack of sexual climax or sex life, can lead on to fibroid tumors, nervous conditions, headaches, tenseness and digestive disorders.

Underlying Negative Mental and Emotional Attitude
Eliminate:
Paying back for the past hurts.
Scared and fearful of
pleasure.
Guilt at recognizing
sexual desires.

Positive Permanent Thinking Replacement
Visualize RED *and repeat:*
My body is full of delight.
I enjoy being a sexual human being.
I revel in the divine gift of union through touch.

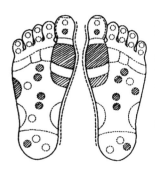

Zone Treatment

Work must be done on all the endocrine system—the pituitary, parathyroids and thyroid glands; also the nervous system, thymus, adrenals, pancreas and ovaries.

Then work on the liver, kidneys and spleen.

<table>
<tr><td>

GALL BLADDER

</td><td>

Healing Color: YELLOW

</td></tr>
</table>

THE area of the body where the gall bladder is, is known as the "Power House". It relates to how good you are at getting your personal needs met. When men and women give up trying to attain their personal power, trouble usually arises in the gall bladder area, stones accumulate or it becomes diseased. If you have never been asked from early life "What would you like?" it's not surprising that this leads to non participation with the human race and constant apathy which will ultimately create a problem in this area, resulting in a need for the organ to be removed later in life. The gall bladder is also connected to the seat of anger, the liver. Great anger will arise from constantly ignoring the "Self" which affects the physical body with bitter bile.

Drink at least six pints of water each day. You need to flush the entire system. Eat plenty of fresh fruit and fresh vegetables. Keep off fatty foods, especially egg yolks, butter, cream and alcohol.

Underlying Negative Mental and Emotional Attitude
Eliminate:
Giving in to bitter thoughts and actions.
Condemning.

Positive Permanent Thinking Replacement
Visualize YELLOW *and repeat:*
I take in only nectar from the gods.
Life is full of sweet honeyed moments.

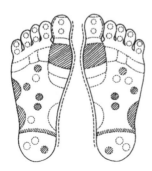

Zone Treatment
Work over the areas in the "Power House'—the gall bladder, liver, kidneys and spleen.

Put pressure too on the thyroids, adrenals, thymus and prostate glands.

Also work on the ascending, descending and sigmoid colons.

GENITAL PROBLEMS

Healing Color: RED

IT is important to flush your bodily systems out completely—drink at least four pints of water a day.

Underlying Negative Mental and Emotional Attitude
Eliminate:
Having sex without love.
Fear of losing sexual charms.
Worried about desirability to the opposite sex or
sexual partner.
Sexual hostage.

Positive Permanent Thinking Replacement
Visualize RED *and repeat:*
I realize all that is unlike love.
I willingly surrender to the exquisite joy
of
sensual fulfillment.

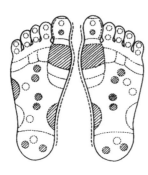

Zone Treatment
Work must be done on the prostate gland for men and the ovaries for women. All that area must be thoroughly massaged.

Then treat the bladder, kidneys, liver, adrenals, thymus, nervous system, thyroids and pituitary glands.

GOUT — Healing Color: GREEN

GOUT is characterized by painful inflammation of certain joints and caused by a build up of acidity.

The first thing you do is to cut out all acidity such as uric acid mostly from red meat, lactic acid such as can be found in whole milk and whole milk products and citric acid from all citrus fruits.

Eat as much green food as you can. As green is alkaline, it combats acidity. Green is a great tonic: it acts upon the system as a cleanser.

Keep off alcohol, especially wines and spirits.

Underlying Negative Mental and Emotional Attitude
Eliminate:
A need to punish the self.
Guilt.
Persecution.

Positive Permanent Thinking Replacement
Visualize GREEN and repeat:
I have the authority to set myself free.
My body vibrates to the excitement of
hope and renewal.

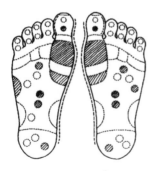

Zone Treatment
Work over the glandular system and organs to eliminate all acidity and toxins. Begin with the liver and kidneys.

Move on to the prostate, adrenals, pancreas, spleen, thymus and pituitary glands.

GUMS

INFLAMED gums, apart from being painful, are extremely unattractive, not to mention the toxic effect that they can have, overloading the glands and creating general constitutional unwellness.

Underlying Negative Mental and Emotional Attitude
Our gums are important to us because they hold our teeth fast.
The teeth need this support because they have the ability to
break down the substance of life.
Eliminate:
You do not support yourself.
The pessimist.

Positive Permanent Thinking Replacement
Visualize BLUE *and repeat:*
I know I can do anything
I want.
I am here for **myself** and
life's purpose.

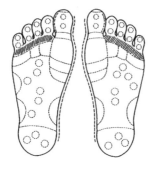

Zone Treatment
The pads under the toes where they join the feet relate to the gum area. Put pressure on this area and work out all tenderness.

HAIR LOSS Healing Color: YELLOW

THERE are many "remedies" and "formulas" for the hair; unfortunately most of them are utter rubbish. The hair is grown from within not without, and your food and the treatment of your body are of paramount importance in the growth of hair. The hair is made up of the same substance as teeth and fingernails, so the reason for hair loss seems to be that not enough of that substance reaches the roots of the hair.

If you wish to have glossy hair, eat plenty of raisins and you will soon begin to see a change in your hair; it will become shiny. Take a lot of vitamin B; all kinds of B vitamins are good for your hair.

It is also a good idea to hold your head down between your knees for a few minutes several times a day. This pressure of the blood to the head stimulates the hair roots. Then you can massage your scalp with your fingertips. Get your fingers on to your scalp and work deeply; also pull and tug the hair. This will loosen your scalp, and allow the blood access to the roots of the hair.

After shampooing your hair, rub glycerine and olive oil in equal parts into your scalp. This treatment will do wonders for your hair.

You may smile at this one, but try it: the nerve endings to the scalp are under your nails so rub your fingernails together for fifteen minutes a day. Do it in three-minute sessions. Buffer the two sets of nails vigorously, you will feel the stimulation.

Underlying Negative Mental and Emotional Attitude Eliminate:
Not allowed to have your own ideas and opinions.
Willful.
Cutting off from creativity.

Positive Permanent Thinking Replacement
Visualize YELLOW *and repeat:*
I can relax and accept my
spontaneity.
I trust my wonderful ideas.

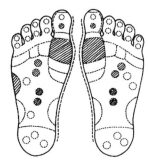

Zone Treatment
Hair loss may indicate that your whole system is under par. Work on the pituitary glands, the thyroid glands, the nervous system, the thymus and adrenal glands, and the liver and kidneys. Work out all tenderness over these areas.

YOU can greatly improve hay fever if you are determined enough. It is most important to correct your breathing. You must never breathe in through your mouth; it must be in through the nose and out through the nose. If you really cannot breathe in through your nose, consult your medical doctor and find out why. Do not breathe into your chest, but breathe deep down into your lower abdomen. Feel your abdomen rush out as you breathe in.

Underlying Negative Mental and Emotional Attitude
Eliminate:
Irritation at the way life is shaping itself.
Fear of changing a belief that **nothing good ever happens.**
My plans get spoilt.
Can't follow through.

Positive Permanent Thinking Replacement
Visualize INDIGO *and repeat:*
I trust I am in the **right place** at the **right time.**
I am part of the **divine plan.**
I have an invitation to the universal party of
LIFE.

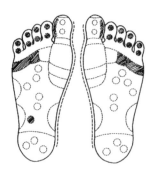

Zone Treatment

You need to treat all areas of membranous tissue. Start by working over all the sinus points, beginning with the big toe. Put pressure on with your fingers and thumbs until you work out all tenderness in those areas. Then go to the points where the toes join the feet, which relate to the eyes and ears, and work all tenderness out there too.

Put pressure on the lungs and chest areas, and the ileocecal valve.

HEADACHES — Healing Color: INDIGO

CONTRARY to what pharmaceutical companies imply by offering one remedy for all associated symptoms, headaches vary widely in their nature, and come from a wide range of causes. Some headaches are relatively dull and throbbing, while others feel sharp or stabbing. Some appear to be nearer the outside of the head, and others are felt deep inside the skull. And they often appear at one side rather than the other, or more towards either front or back.

A headache cannot be dealt with by merely removing the pain, as the drug companies would have us believe. A headache is an indication of stresses affecting other parts of the body, and of our emotional being. Any one of the major organ systems may be linked, as well as factors such as work, home life or relationship. So, treatment of headaches involves working in a way that covers all the most likely causes.

At the same time, we need to eliminate and replace these sources of stress, which we are "opposing" with the headache, rather than resolving. So, while working on the treatment points, we can work on these mental and emotional attitudes, both negative and positive, and simultaneously visualize the associated color, INDIGO.

Underlying Negative Mental and Emotional Attitude
A headache is nature's way of releasing stress through the body from something that is opposing.
Eliminate:
Can't find a way out.
Restrictions.
Constantly criticizing yourself.
Banging your head against a **brick wall**.
Blocked.

I am perfect
just as I am.
Everyone else is perfect, just as they are.
I trust that I can
express myself fully,
in **safety**, and in **peace**.

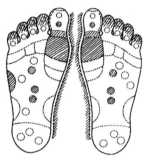

Zone Treatment

Press into each of the top joints in the toes to treat the areas for the eyes and ears. Press along the outside of the big toe and then along the instep of the foot down to the heel; this relates to the whole of the spine.

Work over the points for the pituitary and thyroid glands, nervous system, adrenal glands, liver and kidney. Treat the neck area too—this is at the connection of the big toe to the foot—press both from above and below.

Pay particular attention to whichever of the above points is most painful, as they indicate the body zones that are most relevant to your headache. Over a period of time you may find these particular indications recurring and you will be able to leave out the points and areas that are not relevant for you. For recurring headaches, treat the painful points as often as possible.

For immediate relief treat the roof of the mouth by pressing upwards with your thumb. This stimulates the ear and eye nerves. For headaches on the left, press towards the left side. For those in the middle of the head, press in the centre and so on.

HEART PROBLEMS

Healing Color: GREEN

WITH any sort of heart problem it is important to improve your blood circulation. Try stimulating your legs by using a light wire brush. Stroke up the leg, never down, on both legs, from the ankle upwards. Make the brush strokes light and even.

Underlying Negative Mental and Emotional Attitude
Eliminate:
Problems with love and relationships.
Emotional starvation.
Grieving over **lost love.**

Positive Permanent Thinking Replacement
Visualize GREEN *and repeat:*
The greatest love affair I will ever
have is with my OWN
man or woman within me.
I welcome and embrace this union.

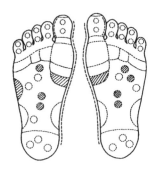

Zone Treatment
You need to work on the main glands and organs in the upper body/chest area. Treat the thymus and adrenal glands, pancreas, liver and kidneys. Massage the heart area with your finger and thumb or a toothbrush handle. Give treatment to all these areas daily.

HEMORRHOIDS — Healing Color: YELLOW

HEMORRHOIDS are caused by painful veins that have become congested; they bleed and often protrude from the anus. They may need surgery. However, using Color Zone Therapy, you can obtain amazing results in improving this complaint.

***Underlying Negative Mental and Emotional Attitude
Eliminate:***
You are blocking yourself off from your true desires.
You cannot take the STRESS of
life
under pressure.

***Positive Permanent Thinking Replacement
Visualize YELLOW and repeat:***
I can remove all blocks and obstacles.
I bring only joy into my life.

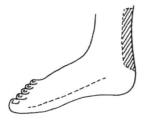

Zone Treatment
Work over the areas up the side of the feet which relate to the rectum. Press firmly—use a toothbrush handle if necessary—to eliminate all soreness.

HEPATITIS

Healing Color: GREEN

HEPATITIS is a disease of the liver. There must be an effort here to purify the bodily system. You must drink at least four pints of good pure water each day. Fruit and vegetables in abundance should be added to your diet; no alcohol at any time.

Underlying Negative Mental and Emotional Attitude
Eliminate:
Anger at being in the **wrong place** at the
wrong time.
A dislike at one's **station** in life.

Positive Permanent Thinking Replacement
Visualize GREEN and repeat:
I trust in universal wisdom.
That I am in the **right place at the right time.**
The world is safe.

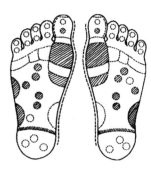

Zone Treatment
Work first on all liver points and kidney points. Then move on to the gall bladder, ascending, sigmoid and descending colons. Give treatment to the pituitary and thyroid glands, nervous system, pancreas, spleen, thymus and adrenal glands. These areas must be massaged until all soreness has been completely eliminated.

HERPES
(Genital)

Healing Color: INDIGO

IF you suffer from this condition, a lot of concentrated work on your part can help you to recover.

Underlying Negative Mental and Emotional Attitude
Eliminate:
Disgust and shame at one's own sexuality.
Sexual guilt.
Revulsion at the self.

Positive Permanent Thinking Replacement
Visualize INDIGO ***and repeat:***
I love and approve of myself.
I am an exquisite
being
by **God's Divine Grace.**

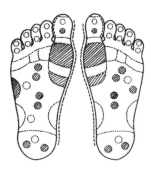

Zone Treatment
The glandular systems must be worked upon hard. Start with the pituitary gland, and then go on to the thyroids, nervous system, thymus, adrenals, pancreas, ovaries or prostate, liver, spleen and kidneys. Give yourself a good treatment until all soreness has completely vanished.

HICCUPS
(or Hiccoughs)

Healing Color: BLUE

IF you suffer from hiccups often, this indicates that you must put your breathing right. Try this breathing exercise. Lie on your back, on a bed or on the floor. Place both hands on your navel, and breathe in to your abdomen rather than the upper chest area, causing your hands to rise. Then breathe out, feeling your hands fall as the abdomen recedes. Continue this for five minutes every day. Make it a habit to drink three or four glasses of pure water each day.

Underlying Negative Mental and Emotional Attitude
Eliminate:
Being UNSETTLED.
I am afraid that I will have to
PERFORM.
People won't accept me the way I am.
I can't COPE—I can't HANDLE it.

Positive Permanent Thinking Replacement
Visualize BLUE and repeat:
As I love and accept others,
others love and accept me.
I can deal with any situation easily and
CALMLY.

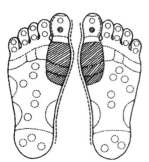

Zone Treatment
Treat the areas for the pituitary and thyroid glands, as well as the areas for the pancreas and stomach.

HIP PROBLEMS   Healing Color: ORANGE

IF your hip problem is an arthritic condition, you can help yourself, depending on how serious it is. In some cases an operation is the only answer, but in most cases Color Zone Therapy can work wonders. Make this treatment a part of your daily life, like brushing your teeth.

Underlying Negative Mental and Emotional Attitude
The pelvic girdle cradles your body. It holds who you are. Hip problems represent no support in **life**.
Eliminate:
Lack of kindness to oneself.

Positive Permanent Thinking Replacement
Visualize ORANGE ***and repeat:***
I am in perfect balance with
myself and the world.
The basin of my body is full of the divine sustenance for
growth.

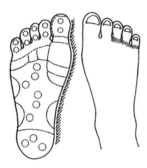

Zone Treatment
Put pressure on all shoulder points, because your shoulders and hips are linked. Work out all tenderness you find. Then cover the entire spinal column. Find all the sore spots in the spine and eliminate them.

On the outside of the ankle, there is a cavity just behind the ankle bone which relates to the hip area (see page 24). Work from the top of that cavity which goes into the leg right down to the bottom of the outside heel. All tenderness must be eliminated.

HOT FLASHES — Healing Color: INDIGO

HOT flashes mean the body is in some kind of change, and that various glands and organs of the body are not working at optimum level. The zone treatment will let you know which these are.

Underlying Negative Mental and Emotional Attitude
Eliminate:
Great rage.
Blocking the flow of progression.
Being afraid of getting old.
Nature has abandoned me.

Positive Permanent Thinking Replacement
Visualize INDIGO and repeat:
I release the need to criticize my
BODY.
I love and ACCEPT myself EXACTLY as I AM.

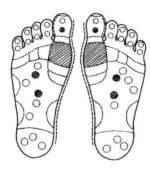

Zone Treatment
The most important areas to treat are those for the pituitary gland—known as the master gland—then the thyroid and adrenal glands, and the nervous system. Press all the points on the feet for the major organs; those that are excessively tender are the ones you need to treat regularly.

IMPOTENCE — Healing Color: ORANGE

THIS distressing condition is, more often than not, caused by emotional and mental rather than physical causes, such as the kind of relationship where partners make life hell for each other over a period of years. In such cases, it is not surprising that "non-performance" occurs. Confidence and self-esteem are shattered, and resentment builds up. However, all is not lost; Color Zone Therapy can certainly help.

Underlying Negative Mental and Emotional Attitude
Eliminate:
Love is scarce.
No beliefs in continuity.
Refusing to recognize nature's sensual signal.
Paying mother back.

Positive Permanent Thinking Replacement
Visualize ORANGE *and repeat:*
I can now release my seeds of LOVE
to bring joy and happiness into the world.

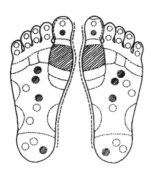

Zone Treatment
It is vitally necessary to be fit and to have your glands functioning at 100 percent. Work over all the endocrine system, beginning with the pituitary glands on each big toe. Then go on to the thyroids, nervous system, thymus, adrenals and prostate glands, and work all tenderness out in all these points.

LOOK at your diet. Good fruit and vegetables are essential. Fresh bananas are especially helpful for this condition.

Underlying Negative Mental and Emotional Attitude Eliminate:
Letting go of one's position in
life.
Fear.

Positive Permanent Thinking Replacement Visualize BLUE *and repeat:*
I trust the process of
life.
I only allow the truth to set me
free.

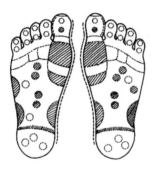

Zone Treatment
Work on bladder, kidneys, liver and spleen. Pay particular attention to the bladder and kidneys. Work away and be determined to eliminate all the sore spots you find. Massage the sigmoid, descending and ascending colons. Then continue to work hard on the pituitary and thyroid glands, nervous system, thymus, pancreas and adrenal glands.

INDIGESTION is usually something only people over twenty-five suffer from. Up to twenty-five most people can eat nails and spit rust and will never suffer from indigestion. But after twenty-five years, the enzyme systems within the pancreatic tract start to malfunction and the older you become the more they malfunction. One answer to this problem is not to eat protein and carbohydrates at the same meal. In most cases, middle age spread is nothing but undigested carbohydrates. So if you follow this discipline, not only do you get rid of your indigestion, but you lose weight as well.

Underlying Negative Mental and Emotional Attitude
Eliminate:
Sour thoughts have entered my system.
I cannot digest them.

Positive Permanent Thinking Replacement
Visualize GREEN *and repeat:*
Life is milk and honey and I will only
absorb and take in
what is good for me.

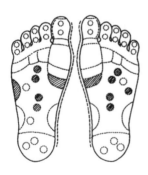

Zone Treatment
The first thing you do is to massage all the pancreas points. All tenderness must be removed. Good pressure is needed; if your fingers and thumbs are too weak, use a toothbrush handle. Move on to the liver, the kidneys, thymus and adrenal glands, and spleen areas. Help ease tension by working on the nervous system.

INFERTILITY
Healing Color: ORANGE

INFERTILITY usually means there is some fault in the endocrine system, that is the reproductive glands. The endocrine glands become unbalanced, meaning a faulty supply of hormones to the system. You should pay special attention to the pituitary, the master gland, for if the pituitary fails to perform, all the other glands in the endocrine system will suffer.

If you think your trouble might be blocked fallopian tubes or a growth on the ovaries, then you must consult your doctor.

Underlying Negative Mental and Emotional Attitude
Eliminate:
Barren thoughts.
No belief in the fruitfulness and gifts of nature.
Not used to receiving.
Fear of being a parent.

Positive Permanent Thinking Replacement
Visualize ORANGE and repeat:
I believe in the spiritual unity through my **physicalness**.
My cup runneth over.
I rejoice in its abundance and **gifts from nature**.

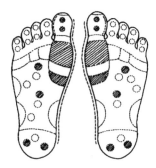

Zone Treatment
Begin with the pituitary gland. All tenderness must be worked out of the pituitary gland areas on both feet. Also treat the thyroid and adrenal glands, and ovaries or prostate. Then massage the thymus and pineal glands, and pancreas. Women should pay special attention to the ovary area. Men need to give special attention to the pituitary.

If your fingers and thumbs are not strong enough use a toothbrush handle. Each day go a little deeper when you give yourself treatment, until all soreness is eliminated.

INFLUENZA

THIS virus will run through you no matter what you do. Once it grabs hold of you, that's it until it decides to leave. It is the aftermath that is most important to deal with, and this is where Color Zone Therapy will really help. The flu will leave every gland and organ in your body feeling as flat as a pancake. This treatment will bring all the glands and organs back up to 100 percent.

Drink at least four pints of good water a day.

Underlying Negative Mental and Emotional Attitude
Eliminate:
Too much going on at once.
Scattered thoughts.
Being pulled in too many directions.
Over scheduled.

Positive Permanent Thinking Replacement
Visualize BLUE and repeat:
I am free to commit to only that
which is important to me.
I can relax.
I shall let my life flow
naturally
with grace and ease.

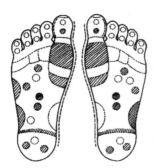

Zone Treatment
Begin with the liver, kidneys, gall bladder and spleen to help purify the system. Then go on to the glandular system. Start with the thyroids, pituitary, thymus, adrenal, pancreas and ovaries or prostate glands. Work the ascending, descending and sigmoid colons.

INSOMNIA

Healing Color: INDIGO

INSOMNIA is often a result of hypertension, anxiety or emotional upset. All these affect the nervous system which in turn affects the glandular system. An overactive thyroid can also keep you awake.

Insomnia becomes habitual after a period of time, for the body clock tunes in to it, so it becomes a difficult habit to break.

A very valuable exercise is to stretch yourself fully out on the bed; relax, and place your thumb in the space between your eyes on your forehead and press. Hold for one minute and relax.

Underlying Negative Mental and Emotional Attitude
Eliminate:
Too afraid to let go of the day.
You must be awake to control events.
Not trusting to surrender.
Suspicious of life's laws.

Positive Permanent Thinking Replacement
Visualize INDIGO *and repeat:*
I can safely let go of the day to become a
beautiful spark knowing that come tomorrow
I shall be me again.

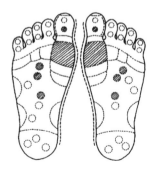

Zone Treatment
The two main glands involved here are the thyroids and the pituitaries. You must work deep into these pressure points. You will feel tenderness, have no doubt, if you suffer from sleeplessness. All this tenderness must be properly worked out. Also massage the nervous system and the thymus and adrenal glands. Then go over the rest of the glandular and organ systems.

JAUNDICE

IF you are unfortunate enough to have suffered from jaundice, you will appreciate how devastating it can be. In terms of Color Zone Therapy, you need the full works here.

You also need to consume plenty of green vegetables and salads. Drink at least four or five pints of water a day and no alcohol.

Underlying Negative Mental and Emotional Attitude
Eliminate:
Feeling unhappy.
Unloved.
Loss of fun in life.
Misplaced confidence.
Not good at pacing
oneself.

Positive Permanent Thinking Replacement
Visualize GREEN *and repeat:*
I rise above all that which is not serving me.
I lift up my hopes.
I glow with supreme confidence and
happiness.

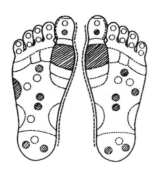

Zone Treatment
Start with the liver and kidneys on the feet first and then on the hands. These two areas are very important for this complaint. Move on to the pituitary, thyroid, thymus and adrenal glands. Massage the spleen and the prostate or ovaries. Work hard and well.

THERE are serious jaw conditions, but here we are dealing with such general matters as the effects of general stress; the jaw is one of the most common places to hold tension, and sometimes there can be a dull ache after grinding the teeth during sleep. Toothache is another source of jaw pain.

Underlying Negative Mental and Emotional Attitude

The jaw shows up strengthened willpower. It becomes painful when there are unexpressed and repressed feelings.

Eliminate:

Repression, unable to express feelings.

No willpower.

Lack of strength.

Deceived.

Positive Permanent Thinking Replacement
Visualize GREEN and repeat:

I will transform I "cannot" into

I "can".

My life is full of brightness.

I move forward with a

merry heart.

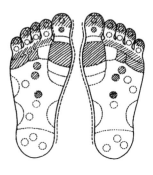

Zone Treatment

Work over all the top joints of the toes. Put the pressure on over those first joints, from the tip down to the joint. All this area must be free from congestion. Next work the pads on the soles, where the toes join the foot—this relates to the jaw area. Massage deep into those pads and eliminate all tenderness. After that, work on the pituitary glands, lungs, chest area, thyroid, nervous system, thymus and adrenal glands.

KIDNEY PROBLEMS

Healing Color: ORANGE

WITH kidney problems, you should consult your medical doctor straight away. But meanwhile, you can also apply Color Zone Therapy without delay.

Underlying Negative Mental and Emotional Attitude
Look at what you might be afraid of, as kidneys react to fear. The adrenal glands are perched on top of the kidneys, ever waiting to go into action to aid us when we go into a "fright and flight" syndrome.
Eliminate:
Unable to face the disappointments and
failures of life.

Positive Permanent Thinking Replacement
Visualize ORANGE *and repeat:*
I have no fear of making mistakes.
Through them I become wise.
They are my greatest opportunity.

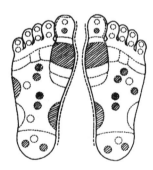

Zone Treatment
Work first of all on all kidney areas. Then work also on the related areas of the bladder, prostate or ovaries, spleen, liver and adrenal glands. Include the thymus, nervous system, thyroids and pituitary glands to help rebalance the body and get the kidneys back to normal functioning.

KNEE PROBLEMS

Healing Color: ORANGE

THE first thing to do is to establish what kind of problem you have with your knee. Is it synovitic water on the knee, is it cartilage or is it plain old arthritis? Whatever condition you have, the treatment of the knee is easy to follow.

Underlying Negative Mental and Emotional Attitude
The knees represent the mechanics of moving forward in life.
Eliminate:
Life is not set up right.
Fear of moving in case you stumble.
Inability to bend with circumstances.

Positive Permanent Thinking Replacement
Visualize ORANGE *and repeat:*
I have no fear of moving forward and being part
of the divine plan.
I do so with **ease** and **grace.**

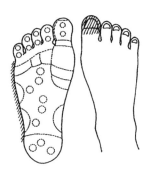

Zone Treatment
To treat the knees, start with the top of the big toe, and work down to the first joint. Clear out any tenderness you may find. Then do the same treatment on the other toes, beginning with the tips and working down to the first joint. Next, look at the sole of the foot; see where the little toe joins it, and on the outside edge massage right down to the outside of the ankle.

LEUKEMIA — Healing Color: YELLOW

LEUKEMIA is caused by a malfunction of the lymphatic system. If you suffer from this condition, you need all the help you can get. If you are unable to do the treatment to yourself, get a member of your family or a good friend to do it for you. Have a treatment every day if possible.

Underlying Negative Mental and Emotional Attitude
Leukemia emotionally signifies the loss of power somewhere so the blood becomes weak and diseased.
Eliminate:
No belief in maturity.
No constant affection.
Betrayed.

Positive Permanent Thinking Replacement
Visualize YELLOW ***and repeat:***
I have the power to
steer my life to
create its potential.
I gain **constant fulfillment**
and **beauty**.

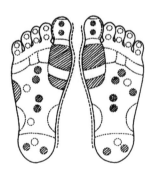

Zone Treatment
The entire glandular and organ systems must be worked upon to enable you to fight the disease. A good idea is to start with the pineal gland then move on to the pituitary gland. Move on to the parathyroids and thyroid glands, and from there go to the nervous systems and thymus. All this takes time so be patient. Massage the adrenals, pancreas, and ovary or prostate regions, from there to the liver, kidneys and spleen.

LIVER COMPLAINTS

Healing Color: GREEN

LIVER conditions can be caused by lots of things; the most common seems to be alcohol. Overindulgence, especially in spirits, will result in a rapid deterioration of the liver. Liquor in moderation is one thing; in excess, it is highly dangerous. Cut out the hard stuff if you want good health.

Underlying Negative Mental and Emotional Attitude
The actual alcohol is not the initial problem. As with all addictions, it is important to find out why you wanted to drink in the first place.
Eliminate:
The liver is the seat of anger.
It absorbs and takes the brunt of all our **experiences**.
Can be **self-deception**.

Positive Permanent Thinking Replacement
Visualize GREEN ***and repeat:***
I am ready and prepared.
I trust that whatever **comes my way**
is **given** to me with **love** by the **world**.

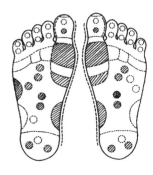

Zone Treatment
Start with the kidneys; these must function strongly to help you avoid infection. Then move on to the liver and gall bladder. Go on to the adrenal, pancreas and thymus glands, nervous system, pituitary, thyroid, ovaries or prostate glands, and bladder. Work with determination on all of the areas, and keep right on working until all tenderness has been eliminated completely.

Healing Color: INDIGO

LUMBAGO affects the lower back. It can be treated success-fully. If you're prepared to work at it, the results can be excellent. Practice your treatment at any time you can.

Underlying Negative Mental and Emotional Attitude
Eliminate:
Aiming too low in life.
Stooping.
Being put upon.
A martyr.
Back-breaking beliefs.

Positive Permanent Thinking Replacement
Visualize INDIGO *and repeat:*
I can lift myself up into the hills
from whence my help comes.
I feel **wonderful**.
Tall and towering.

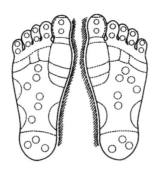

Zone Treatment
Massage all the lower back area and the hip area. Then work up the entire spinal column. Work until all tenderness has been eliminated.

LUNG TROUBLES

Healing Color: INDIGO

IF you suffer from lung or bronchial trouble and you smoke, you should give it up without delay. Always try to breathe in and out through your nose, not your mouth. Breathe deep down into the abdomen, as low as you can. Practice this daily. Visualize your healing color, INDIGO, especially during your breathing exercises, until it becomes part of you.

Underlying Negative Mental and Emotional Attitude
Eliminate:

Have not experienced the "give" and "take" of life.
The fear of being unwanted and abandoned.
Unable to accept that which
cannot be changed.

Positive Permanent Thinking Replacement
Visualize INDIGO and repeat:

It is safe for me to
**expand my horizons and
spread my wings**.

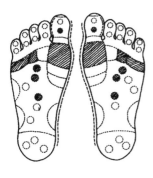

Zone Treatment

Start by massaging all the lung and chest areas. This work must be done in a dedicated way until all soreness has been eliminated. Then proceed to the nervous system, thymus, adrenal, thyroids and pituitary glands. Work with a will and show determination. Have total faith and commitment and good results will manifest.

MENOPAUSE · Healing Color: ORANGE

PROBLEMS associated with menopause can include hot flushes, being nervous or panicky, being spaced out, just not feeling well: so what can be done? One treatment is hormone replacement therapy (HRT), which is also a safeguard against osteoporosis. However, HRT does not suit everyone. The Color Zone Therapy for this condition is very effective.

Underlying Negative Mental and Emotional Attitude
In ancient tribes it was not the young woman who was the most revered, but the older, wise woman, who was always past her menopause. The belief was that when menstruation ceased, then a woman was really gifted with maturity and divine creativity.

Eliminate:
Battering against the **tide** of **time**.
Convinced that nature has **abandoned me**.
A **fear** that I won't be wanted any more.
Redundant.

Positive Permanent Thinking Replacement
Visualize orange *and repeat:*
I trust the process of life.
I release the old and **welcome the new**.
I thank the universe for its process and wisdom,
I am happy to take my place in its **wondrous plan** of **constant renewal**.

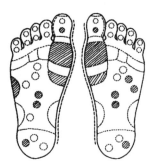

Zone Treatment
Work on the pituitary, thyroid and adrenal glands, pancreas and ovaries, taking all the soreness out of those areas. Then tone up the liver, kidneys, heart and spleen. Give yourself a twenty-minute treatment each day.

MENSTRUAL PAIN

Healing Color: INDIGO

START your work about five days before your period begins, and keep giving yourself the treatment until your period begins.

You could also incorporate this simple exercise. Sit on the floor with your legs open as wide apart as they will go, and gently rock your body forwards and backwards. Your arms remain loosely by your side while you keep this gentle rocking movement up, for at least five minutes. It's very good to work on just before a period begins, as it helps to decongest the pelvic area.

You should also treat the whole of your reproductive system.

Underlying Negative Mental and Emotional Attitude Eliminate:
It's no good being female.
A belief that women must suffer.
Would rather be a little girl.
Don't want to grow up.

Positive Permanent Thinking Replacement Visualize INDIGO *and repeat:*
I can enjoy and relax in the rhythm and flow of **life**.
I welcome the **red snow** of **refreshment**.

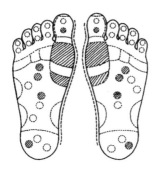

Zone Treatment
Work on the thyroid and pituitary glands, nervous system, thymus, pancreas, adrenal glands and ovaries. Take a large spoon and use the handle to put pressure on your tongue. Pay particular attention to the middle of the tongue, going from the tip to as far back as possible. This connects directly to the womb and the ovaries. Start with a one-minute treatment on the tongue and each day add a few seconds until you are up to three minutes.

MIGRAINE — Healing Color: INDIGO

THERE is a lot that you can do for yourself with migraine headaches. You should check your diet first. It has been found that by eliminating certain foods that can trigger off an attack, you will be able to bring about some relief. These include chocolate, hard cheeses, citrus fruits, alcohol, over-ripe bananas, raspberries and fried fatty foods. Once you have become careful with what you eat, you can bring in the Color Zone approach.

Underlying Negative Mental and Emotional Attitude
Eliminate:
Frustrations at not being free to express desires.
Bottled up emotions exploding.
Being driven against your will.

Positive Permanent Thinking Replacement
Visualize INDIGO and repeat:
From now on I shall take **control** of **my life** and work in unity so that I can **live**, **laugh** and **love** in my **own time**.

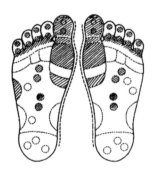

Zone Treatment
First of all, massage all the sinus points. Then work under the big toe from where it joins the foot, right to the tip of the toe. This area relates to the neck. You must use quite a bit of pressure; if necessary use the handle of a toothbrush.

Next, work across the top of the feet where the toes join the foot, from the back of the big toe right across to the little toe. See that your fingernails are cut short, then work as deeply as you can over that area. Then work on all eye and ear points. Finally massage the pituitary and thyroid glands, nervous system, thymus and adrenal glands, pancreas, liver and kidneys.

WITH MS, you can do a lot to help yourself in the early stages if you are of a positive mind, for this condition responds to positiveness. You cannot afford to sit back and accept it; that's fatal. You must be determined to help yourself, to retain as near normal health as possible. Color Zone Therapy can help you to do just that. Try to practice it on a daily basis.

Underlying Negative Mental and Emotional Attitude
Eliminate:
A belief in the underdog.
Spirit weakened.
Can't do it. It's too much for me.

Positive Permanent Thinking Replacement
Visualize INDIGO and repeat:
I can now take charge of my life because
I love and approve of myself.
I am forever powerful.

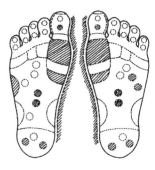

Zone Treatment
Follow the line of points for the spinal column up from the bottom of the heel, taking in the coccyx, the sacrum and the lumbar area. Work out all soreness. Then work on all glands and organs— the pituitary, thyroid, pancreas, adrenal and ovaries or prostate glands, heart, spleen, liver and kidneys.

MYALGIC ENCEPHALO-MYELITIS (ME)

Healing Color: YELLOW

COMMON symptoms for this distressing condition include excessive and constant weakness and fatigue, persistent muscle pain, lack of concentration, headaches, giddiness and painful joints. ME can be treated successfully with Color Zone Therapy, if you work with determination and persistence.

Underlying Negative Mental and Emotional Attitude
Eliminate:
Muddled energies – muddled thinking.
Unable to take control.
UNCONNECTED.

Positive Permanent Thinking Replacement
Visualize YELLOW *and repeat:*
I am what I am.
It's great to be
ME.
It's great to be
M.E.

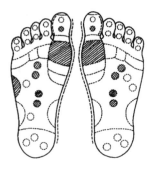

Zone Treatment
The state of the thyroid gland seems to be a key factor in this condition, so work especially on this. Then work on the pituitary, thymus and adrenal glands, and nervous system to boost your whole system. Finally work on the liver and kidneys.

NAUSEA

MOST nausea that occurs regularly is caused by hyper-glycemia, brought on by low blood sugar. If you suffer from this, you must eat some good quality fruit or protein every two to three hours. The most important organs concerned are the pancreas and spleen, but the liver, kidneys and stomach are also involved.

Underlying Negative Mental and Emotional Attitude
Eliminate:
Feeling a failure.
Sick of being put upon.
CAN'T do it.
Feeling HUMILIATED.

Positive Permanent Thinking Replacement
Visualize GREEN and repeat:
I shall not hide from the
WORLD.
I now go beyond all fears and limitations.
I release the past with
LOVE.

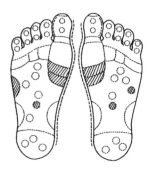

Zone Treatment
Treat the areas for the pancreas and spleen. Then treat the areas for the liver, kidneys and stomach. Work between the big toes and second toes, deep into the 'valley' between. This area relates to the stomach.

It can also be helpful to treat the corresponding area on each hand, pressing into the valley between the thumb and index finger.

THERE are many forms of nervous conditions, including phobias. What sufferers have in common is that they are all looking for peace of mind, tranquillity, contentment and happiness. To overcome a nervous disorder takes some doing, but it can be done with determination, faith and single-mindedness.

The first thing to do is to practice the healing treatment. Lie down, stretch out completely, relax, put both hands on your stomach, fingertips just touching, breathe in, hold for four seconds and breathe out. Do this exercise frequently for one week. Then add one count and do five in, hold for five and five out. Each week add one count until you are doing ten in, hold for ten and ten out. All breathing must be done through the nose, never use the mouth.

All the time you are doing your breathing exercise, you must visualize the healing color, YELLOW. You will find after a little time that you are becoming calmer and more peaceful.

If you suffer from a nervous condition, you need a lot of courage, desire and will to overcome it, but you can do it if you really want to. You have a lot to do; you must generate the energy to work at getting better.

Underlying Negative Mental and Emotional Attitude
Eliminate:
The nerves are like the telephone exchange.
The receivers and communicators.
Nervous disorders show a breakdown in the junction box in the
receptive department.
FEAR.

Positive Permanent Thinking Replacement
Visualize YELLOW and repeat:
I love the networking in my body of love and light.
I look forward to its **clear messages.**

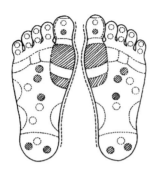

Zone Treatment

Nervous disorders can be helped by working on your thyroid and pituitary glands. Work on the nervous system, thymus, adrenal, pancreas and ovaries or prostate glands. You must work away until all soreness has been eliminated.

IF you experience this problem, the first thing to do is to visit your dentist; generally speaking, if your teeth are in good order, you shouldn't suffer from neuralgia. However, when you are run down, stress can show up as neuralgic pain.

Underlying Negative Mental and Emotional Attitude
Only one kind of worry is proper: to worry because you worry so much.
Eliminate:
Unsolved worries.
Self-limiting.
Fear of humiliation.

Positive Permanent Thinking Replacement
Visualize INDIGO and repeat:
I have no need of **approval** from others.
I approve of my **divine place** in this
world.

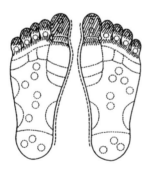

Zone Treatment
Begin by working on the top joints of the toes with your fingers and thumbs, and gradually work down to the first joint. Do this on all the toes to stimulate all the zones. Apply pressure to the pads on the soles, just below where the toes join the foot. After that, massage all the glands and organs, for you need a good general tone-up.

NUMBNESS

ON the whole, numbness is a temporary phenomenon, usually caused by poor circulation; if it is persistent, you should definitely consult a doctor. In addition to the treatment given below, try this exercise. Take a soft wire brush and brush upwards, never downwards, from where the toes join the top of the foot. Brush upwards from the toes to the ankle on the top of the foot, and then repeat the performance from the sole of the foot up to the ankle. Do twenty strokes each session.

Underlying Negative Mental and Emotional Attitude
Eliminate:
A cutting off from feelings.
A turning off of unpleasant situations.
Cannot believe what is going on in environment.
Deciding to quit.

Positive Permanent Thinking Replacement
Visualize YELLOW and repeat:
I choose to switch on to the
new and **exciting experience that life holds for me**.
Every day and in **every way** I become **stronger** and **stronger**.

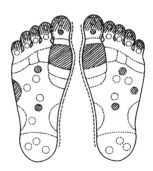

Zone Treatment
Pressurize the tips of the toes to stimulate all the zones, then work over all the top joints.

Massage the liver and kidneys. Move on to your spleen, thymus, thyroid and pituitary glands, making sure that all soreness has been eliminated from all areas.

PARKINSON'S DISEASE

Healing Color: GREEN

AT the moment there is no known cure for Parkinson's disease. But it can be helpful for the patient to have every gland and organ in the body working as well as possible. It would be better to encourage another member of your family or a friend to give the zone treatment to you; you need a lot of vigor and energy put into it so that you will really feel the benefits. You need a lot of faith here, too, but you can help yourself a lot, especially in the early stages of the disease.

Underlying Negative Mental and Emotional Attitude Eliminate:
Lost confidence with life.
Life is never certain.
Fearful of change.

Positive Permanent Thinking Replacement
Visualize GREEN *and repeat:*
The most beautiful thing that
I can experience is the
mystery.
I **rejoice** in **life's**
opportunities.

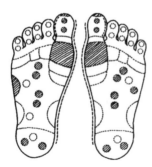

Zone Treatment
Start work on the brain, pineal and pituitary glands, the thyroids, the nervous system, thymus, adrenal and prostate or ovary glands. Then move on to the liver, kidneys and spleen.

PROSTATE PROBLEMS	Healing Color: YELLOW (to increase flow) Healing Color: INDIGO (to decrease flow)

THIS condition affects most men over fifty years of age. It mostly affects performance when attempting to urinate; either you are going every ten minutes, it seems, or else you can find it difficult to urinate at all. This is because the gland is swollen, and is affecting the bladder.

Treatment with Color Zone Therapy is fairly easy—it can and does help prostate trouble. If you work hard and conscientiously, you will be really amazed at the results you will obtain.

Underlying Negative Mental and Emotional Attitude
Eliminate:
Afraid to let go of the **identity** of
being **macho**.
Feeling less than a man.
Fear of the future because of aging.

Positive Permanent Thinking Replacement
Visualize YELLOW *or* INDIGO *and repeat:*
I am youth and joy.
I know the **cosmos motivates** at all **levels**.
I enter this time of my life with
expectations of complete harmony
with myself and my surroundings.
I **allow** the **sunlight** to **enter** my **soul**.

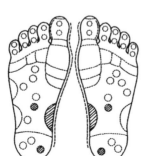

Zone Treatment
Work upon the areas marked for the prostate. Also pay attention to the bladder and kidney areas.

PYORRHEA

Healing Color: BLUE

THIS is an inflammation of the gums. In this condition, you are definitely run down and badly need to be picked up, so a comprehensive type of treatment is required.

Underlying Negative Mental and Emotional Attitude
Deep-rooted disturbances in the family from early childhood.

Eliminate:
Resentment at having to live
life this way.
Always going down the
wrong track.

Positive Permanent Thinking Replacement
Visualize BLUE ***and repeat:***
I can transplant my ideas any time.
I'm in the right place at the right time.
I trust that only the right action will take place in my life.

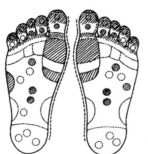

Zone Treatment
All the top joints of the toes have to be treated. Keep the pressure on for thirty seconds, then rest, followed by another thirty seconds. Notice how the toes join the soles, and put pressure on all the pads just underneath, where the toes join the feet. This is the jaw and gum area.

Then work on all major glands such as the pituitary, thyroids, pancreas, adrenal and thymus. Continue on to the liver, spleen and kidneys. Work all eye zones.

SCIATICA

Healing Color: INDIGO

THIS is an extremely painful condition that starts in the hip and can run down the leg, even to the back of the heel. It is usually due to the sciatic nerve being trapped and inflamed. It will respond well to Color Zone Therapy, as well as to rest and heat.

Underlying Negative Mental and Emotional Attitude
Eliminate:
Out of depth.
Traumatic events have been happening.

Positive Permanent Thinking Replacement
Visualize INDIGO ***and repeat:***
I am now sailing into
smooth waters.
I feel **cool, calm** and
collected.

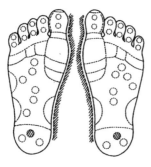

Zone Treatment
Work on the outside of the heel all around the ankle bone and up the side of the foot into the cavity there. Get rid of all the soreness. Deeply massage the sciatic nerve points on the heel pads with a toothbrush handle. Then the area for the bottom of the spine must be massaged, and up the ankle, on the inside of the foot. Then proceed and work up the entire spinal column. In those areas you will find all the nerves to the sciatica.

SHINGLES

Healing Color: GREEN

THIS condition is a difficult one, and dealing with it requires a lot of patience. You will be very run down and anxious. But if you are prepared to work at it, you will see a positive result. Have faith in your ability to succeed.

Underlying Negative Mental and Emotional Attitude
Eliminate:
Constant reminder of **past hurts**.
Not wanting to face reality.
Living in a fool's paradise.

Positive Permanent Thinking Replacement
Visualize GREEN *and repeat:*
I release all past sorrows.
I trust the process of renewal.
All is being made
safe and clear for me.

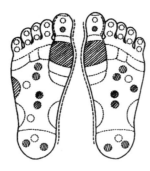

Zone Treatment
The first things to work upon are the nervous system, the thyroid glands, the thymus and the adrenal glands. You must eliminate all tenderness from these areas. Then massage the liver, kidneys and spleen, and from there to the pituitary, and ovaries or prostate glands.

SINUSITIS is an infection, which can be mild or extreme. In order to cut down on mucus within the system, cut out all milk products, including butter and cheese, and also eggs. Sinus trouble responds well to Color Zone Therapy; while continuing the procedures below, you can also use inhalants, steam inhalation under a towel, and vapor rub.

Underlying Negative Mental and Emotional Attitude
Eliminate:
Uncried tears from **childhood**.
No **structure** within the **family** from early age.

Positive Permanent Thinking Replacement
Visualize INDIGO and repeat:
I am not alone.
I **love** my little child within me;
whatever happens I am always here for
him or **her**.

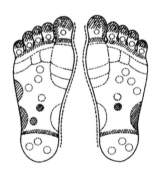

Zone Treatment
Massage the main sinus points on the big toes. Then massage the top joints of the toes, from the big toe to the little toe. Put pressure on all the pads of the feet just under the toes, on the soles. Work on the liver and kidneys, the ileo-cecal valve, the ascending colon, sigmoid colon and the descending colon to help purify the system.

SKIN PROBLEMS

Healing Color: YELLOW

MOST skin conditions are deep-seated, and can be caused through the body being allergic, perhaps to certain foods, to drink, to emotional issues, or to the air that you breathe. So it may also be worth consulting the treatments for Allergies and for Emotional Problems. Skin conditions respond strongly to treatment for the glands, especially the adrenals, thyroid and pituitary. It is also important to treat the liver and its associated organ, the gall bladder; also the kidneys.

Underlying Negative Mental and Emotional Attitude Eliminate:
Cannot be assertive.
Constant eruptions.
IRRITATION.
Unresolved problems with past parental upsets.
Lack of the consistency of unconditional
LOVE.

Positive Permanent Thinking Replacement Visualize YELLOW *and repeat:*
I comfort my inner child and we are safe.
I'm confident in expressing my feelings.
I am focused.
I deserve the best in everything.

Zone Treatment

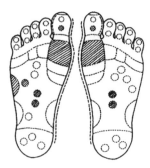

Treat the areas for the adrenal, thyroid and pituitary glands. Find which of these points are the tender ones, and focus your work on them—these will be the glands that are malfunctioning in your particular condition. Also treat the areas relating to the liver, gall bladder and kidneys to ensure any impurities are eliminated from your system.

SPONDYLITIS & STIFF NECK

SPONDYLITIS is an arthritic condition of the neck, which is painful and limits movement. The first thing to do is cut out all acidity such as uric acid (red meat), lactic acid (dairy products) and citric acid (citrus fruits). Twice a day, take cider vinegar and honey; mix a tablespoon of cider vinegar and a tablespoon of honey in equal portions in a cup, add warm water, stir and drink. Also take a tablespoonful of black molasses each day, mixed with warm water.

Underlying Negative Mental and Emotional Attitude
Eliminate:
Rigidity of thought.
Fear of going with the flow.
Inflexible.
Stubborn.

Positive Permanent Thinking Replacement
Visualize INDIGO *and repeat:*
I can twist, turn and bend with the
flow of life.
I am a moving miracle.

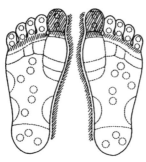

Zone Treatment
Work all the neck area, especially where the big toe joins the foot. Start from the joint and work up into the big toe. Do the same on the back of the big toe, and massage across the top of the foot from the big toe to the little toe where the toes join the foot. Also massage the area for the entire spinal column. Also follow the treatment for arthritis to help eliminate acidity from the body.

FOR stomach problems, eat plenty of greenery and fresh fruit. Drink four or more pints of water a day. Give yourself at least twenty minutes of the treatment described, each day.

Underlying Negative Mental and Emotional Attitude
This area absorbs and takes the brunt of all experiences.
Eliminate:
Unable to take in the nutrients of
life.
Can't stomach the situation.
Not good at nurturing
oneself.

Positive Permanent Thinking Replacement
Visualize GREEN *and repeat:*
I can take all that is
NEW
and allow it to give me
love and comfort in peace.

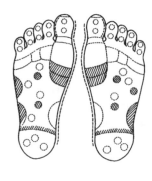

Zone Treatment
Begin by pressurizing the descending colon, sigmoid colon and ascending colon. Then work on the rest of the digestive system, the liver, kidneys, spleen, stomach area and pancreas. Also treat the nervous system. Work all the tenderness out of those areas. Then take a large spoon and with the handle of the spoon put pressure over the tongue. Do all this on a daily basis. This will bring relief to the stomach area.

FOR internal ulcers, always consult your medical practitioner, then add the Color Zone Therapy.

Underlying Negative Mental and Emotional Attitude Eliminate:
Not acknowledged in any areas of life.
Frustration.
A belief that one can only be loved for what one does, and not for who one is.
Extreme irritation.

Positive Permanent Thinking Replacement Visualize GREEN *and repeat:*
I can see the green fields of home.
This place is mine, and the universe knows it.
It is just fine to ease myself into deep rest.

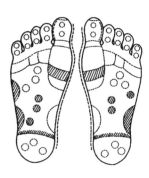

Zone Treatment
Work upon the stomach, kidneys and liver, the adrenal glands, spleen and ileocecal valve. Also, treat the ascending, descending and sigmoid colons.

STRESS & STRAIN

Healing Color: BLUE

STRESS seems to be the bottom line in most conditions, and in itself can become very serious indeed if neglected. It undermines the physical, emotional and mental bodies. Peace of mind, contentment and tranquillity are yearned for by people who suffer from stress. If stress is your problem, you must balance your entire being back to perfection; always practice your Color Zone Therapy every day.

Underlying Negative Mental and Emotional Attitude
Eliminate:
Not good at pacing oneself.
Unable to divide life up into
work and play.
Lack of self-discipline.

Positive Permanent Thinking Replacement
Visualize BLUE *and repeat:*
I can relax **knowing** that
at the end of the day
I have done the **best**
I can.
Tomorrow is another day.

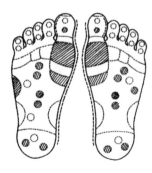

Zone Treatment
Begin work over the thyroid gland and nervous system. Move on to the pituitary glands, then to the thymus and adrenal glands, pancreas and spleen. All soreness must be completely eliminated from these areas.

Pressure must then be put on to the liver, kidneys and ovaries or prostate. You need to get all your glands and organs back to 100 percent.

ULTIMATELY, stroke is the result of anxiety and stress. It usually occurs when high blood pressure causes a blood clot in the brain. Nervous impulses to the side of the body affected cannot be transmitted and the muscles become paralyzed. To prevent stroke, and to deal with it, you must become a non-worrier. The key organ is the pituitary gland, but it is helpful to work over the other glands and the major organs as well. It is important to start work as soon as possible after the stroke. A friend or relative will need to do the treatment for you.

Underlying Negative Mental and Emotional Attitude Eliminate:
Not counting.
Afraid of dying.
In one stroke, one can remove oneself from the world.
Don't want to be a
BURDEN.

Positive Permanent Thinking Replacement
Visualize YELLOW *and repeat:*
I trust the process of life.
I will always **ATTRACT** the help I need.
I am on an **ENDLESS JOURNEY** through **ETERNITY.**

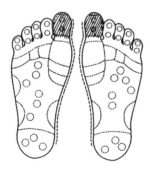

Zone Treatment
Treat the area for the pituitary gland and continue working over all areas of the big toe. The top of this toe represents the brain. Massage from the top down to the root, including the sides and back of the toe. Concentrate most on the toe which is on the opposite side of the body to the side affected. If possible, also press all the other major treatment points for organs and glands.

STUTTER & STAMMER

Healing Color: BLUE

YOU have approximately sixty muscles in your throat and they all need exercising. You will find the following helpful if you tend to stammer and stutter. Open your mouth and sing up a scale. Practice singing instead of talking. If you are really willing to do these exercises, you will be surprised at the results.

Underlying Negative Mental and Emotional Attitude
Eliminate:
Persecuted.
A belief that words don't count.
Words can be false and treacherous.
Rather not say them.
Unsure that it will be understood.

Positive Permanent Thinking Replacement
Visualize BLUE *and repeat:*
My words are
sweet music to
my ears.
I flow easily with the rhythm of speech from the
purity of my heart.

Zone Treatment
Take a dry napkin or towel. Put your tongue out, take hold of it with the napkin, and pull your tongue out in little jerks. As you do so, also move your tongue to the right and to the left, and then clockwise and counterclockwise. Do this for a minute; have a little rest, and then repeat. Do this four or five times a day.

THRUSH (CANDIDA)

Healing Color: GREEN

THRUSH can be an extremely debilitating condition, almost like a torture. You will be feeling very run down. If you suffer from this, it is advisable to stay off dairy products.

Underlying Negative Mental and Emotional Attitude
Eliminate:
Feeling abused as a woman.
Not happy with partner.
Anger.

Positive Permanent Thinking Replacement
Visualize GREEN *and repeat:*
I am the **passage** to **bliss.**
I love and **rejoice** in my
female sexuality.

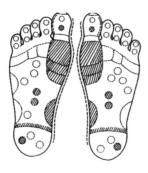

Zone Treatment
A lot of work must be done on the urinary system, the bladder, kidneys, anus and vagina areas; eliminate all tenderness in those regions. Massage the ovaries, the stomach, the sigmoid colon, adrenal, pancreas and thyroid glands. Work on the pituitary gland to help boost your whole system.

THYROID

OVERACTIVE
UNDERACTIVE

Healing Color: BLUE
Healing Color: ORANGE

THE Zone Therapy treatments for these two conditions are the same, but the healing colors are different. For an overactive thyroid you must use BLUE, for an underactive thyroid use ORANGE. Be prepared to have the patience and determination to gain the rewards you are seeking.

Underlying Negative Mental and Emotional Attitude
Eliminate:
A belief that if one keeps moving one will be out of danger (for the overactive thyroid).
Restrictions in life (for the underactive thyroid).
What's the use of balance?
A fear of **old age** and **death**.
A giving up of normality.

Positive Permanent Thinking Replacement
Visualize BLUE or ORANGE and repeat:
I will no longer **sabotage** myself.
I will make the most of all that **comes** and
the **least of that which goes**.

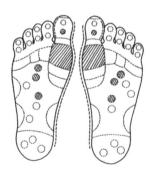

Zone Treatment
Begin by massaging the parathyroids and thyroid glands. Do this thoroughly. Then massage the nervous system, the thymus, adrenal and pituitary glands.

TINNITUS

TINNITUS involves experiencing continuous ringing and noise in the ears; it can be very wearing to the whole system. It indicates a deterioration of the middle ear.

Underlying Negative Mental and Emotional Attitude
Eliminate:
Wilfulness.
Determined not to hear.
Prefer one's **own sound** to the
noise of life.

Positive Permanent Thinking Replacement
Visualize YELLOW and repeat:
I can hear, in more ways than one, the
universal sounds.
I trust I shall receive **harmonious** keys for life's
adventures.

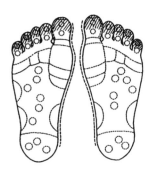

Zone Treatment
Work over the top joint of the toes, paying particular attention to the third and fourth toes which relate to the ears. Eliminate all soreness.

After that, work on the entire glandular system.

TRAVEL SICKNESS

Healing Color: GREEN

IF you suffer from car, sea or air sickness, you need treatment for your organs of balance. The fault lies in the ears and eyes, and you need to pay attention to the ears first.

Underlying Negative Mental and Emotional Attitude
Eliminate:
Fear of moving from one place to another.
Afraid to be alone.

Positive Permanent Thinking Replacement
Visualize GREEN and repeat while travelling:
I shall take each second
one at a time;
I am **safe** this second.
I am safe from one second to another.

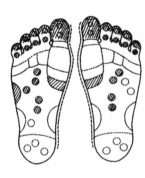

Zone Treatment
Work over all the toes, paying particular attention to the end toes. Do all the points marked for the ears, very thoroughly. Work all the tenderness out of the big toes especially. Then work over the liver, kidneys, gall bladder, nervous system, thymus and adrenal glands, and pancreas. Next, give treatment to all the eye nerves. Work out all tenderness appertaining to the eyes.

TUBERCULOSIS — Healing Color: INDIGO

IN the 1990s TB is beginning to rear its ugly head again—in the mid 1950s the clinics for its treatment were closed down, as it had been controlled.

Underlying Negative Mental and Emotional Attitude Eliminate:
Fearful.
Feeling victimized.
Negative thoughts eating away at life's energy.
No belief in give and **take**.

Positive Permanent Thinking Replacement Visualize INDIGO *and repeat:*
I acknowledge that peace and harmony
dwell within me.
I can seize each day with
joy and excitement.

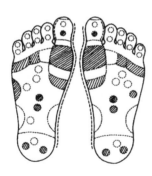

Zone Treatment
Massage the lungs and chest areas. Also pay attention to the liver and kidneys. Then work upon the glands of the thyroid and pituitary, the pancreas, adrenals, spleen and prostate or ovaries.

URINARY INFECTIONS

Healing Color: INDIGO

THIS condition is distressing and painful, and also embarrassing due to the frequent need to empty the bladder. Such infections must not be ignored, as they can affect the kidneys, so you should contact your doctor if the condition is persistent.

Underlying Negative Mental and Emotional Attitude
Eliminate:
Weakened by circumstances.
Rushing around for **others**.
Can't hold on much longer.

Positive Permanent Thinking Replacement
Visualize INDIGO *and repeat:*
I will no longer do things at the
expense of **myself.**
I **release** all that is **not**
serving me.

Zone Treatment

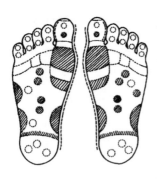

Begin by massaging the bladder and the kidneys on the left foot; remove all the soreness out of those areas. Then start to work on the sigmoid, ascending and descending colons. Put pressure on the liver and kidney points, after which you can massage the spleen, pancreas, adrenal, thymus, nervous system, thyroid and pituitary glands.

VARICOSE VEINS

Healing Color: INDIGO

THE main cause of varicose veins is the liver which is failing to process the blood correctly, resulting in clots. If your varicose veins are new, you can help them a great deal with this treatment. If they are very bad, then you should see a varicose vein specialist.

Underlying Negative Mental and Emotional Attitude
Eliminate:
Stagnation.
Stuck in situations of long standing that you
dislike.

Positive Permanent Thinking Replacement
Visualize INDIGO *and repeat:*
I can move freely from place to place in my
heart and the **universe**.

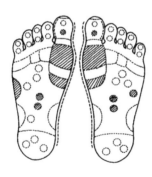

Zone Treatment
You must begin by working on the liver, removing all soreness from the liver area. Next are the kidneys and spleen; work well on these points.

After that, tone up the adrenal, pancreas, thyroid and pituitary glands. If you find the treatment hard to do with your fingers, use a toothbrush handle.

VERTIGO

Healing Color: INDIGO

IF you suffer from vertigo, you must have your ears and also eyes checked by a medical specialist; it is usually the middle ear that is problematic. The state of the sinuses is also closely related to this problem.

Underlying Negative Mental and Emotional Attitude
Eliminate:
Uncommitted.
Unable to stand up for oneself.
People don't accept one.
Afraid of being sick, and unable to take care of oneself.

Positive Permanent Thinking Replacement
Visualize INDIGO and repeat:
I am very
SPECIAL.
I am who I am, and I state my needs and wants,
easily and effortlessly.
What I am counts in this
WORLD.
I deserve the best in
EVERYTHING.

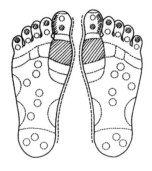

Zone Treatment
Work strongly on the areas for the sinuses. Also treat the areas for the pituitary and thyroid glands. Check all the other glands and organs; if any of these are particularly tender, there is congestion contributing to your condition, so those points should be added to your daily treatment.

VITALITY (LACK OF)

Healing Color: RED

IF you suffer from poor vitality, you must be sure you take the correct vitamins. Vitamin B12 is the most important, together with all the B vitamins, as well as vitamins E and A. Also, start to take brewers' yeast on a daily basis. You may also need extra iron. If you suffer from poor vitality, there must be a reason for it. Color Zone Therapy will help you deal with the causes.

Underlying Negative Mental and Emotional Attitude
Eliminate:
Fear of success.
Sorrows.
Lack interest in life and
surroundings.

Positive Permanent Thinking Replacement
Visualize RED and repeat:
The world is continually offering me gifts of
life.
I willingly accept the
opportunities
with **fun and joy**.

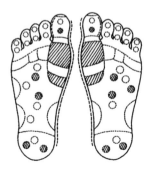

Zone Treatment
Start with the pituitary glands; then move on to the glands of the thyroid, adrenal, pancreas, ovaries or prostate and nervous system.

Also treat the spleen, which will be particularly affected if you are short of iron. You have to eliminate all tenderness from your feet.

WATER RETENTION

THERE are few things more uncomfortable than the bloated feeling and general malaise that this condition brings on—not to mention clothes not fitting any more! Water retention can be a lymphatic problem, or it can be due to a malfunction of the kidneys or bladder.

Underlying Negative Mental and Emotional Attitude
Eliminate:
Internal body tears.
Not trusting to let go.
A banking up of old ideas.
Blocked.

Positive Permanent Thinking Replacement
Visualize YELLOW and repeat:
I am **free** to go as I **please**.
I **welcome** life's **changes**.
I welcome and relax into the
beloved circles
that are taking place in my
LIFE.

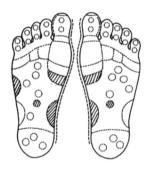

Zone Treatment
You must work on the bladder and kidney areas on both hands and feet. Pay particular attention to the lymph glands (see page 24), for you must eliminate all tenderness from this area, too. Also, work upon the liver and pancreas.

WEIGHT PROBLEMS
(OVERWEIGHT)

Healing Color: YELLOW

THERE is no mystery about losing weight if you are in normal health. Unless you suffer from an underactive thyroid or some metabolic problem, being overweight means you are eating too much or, worse still, you are loading up with junk food; most weight problems in those over twenty-five years of age are due to undigested carbohydrates. You eat protein specially to build up muscle, and carbohydrates for energy. If you are not digesting your carbohydrates, they become undigested body fat, useless for your bodily needs.

The answer is simple. Never, unless you are obliged to, eat protein and carbohydrates at the same meal. Make a rule: one meal carbohydrates, the next meal protein. So when you eat protein, such as meat or fish, do not eat bread, potatoes, rice or pasta at the same time. With either protein or carbohydrates, you can eat all the greenery and fruit you want. Don't eat chocolate biscuits, sweets and cakes at all.

Underlying Negative Mental and Emotional Attitude
Fat is fear. Continued fear causes a person to be fat and weak.
There is a lack of firmness in the person's life.
Eliminate:
Fear of being noticed.
Unable to be your real self.
Can't get needs met.
Avoiding sexuality.

Positive Permanent Thinking Replacement
Visualize YELLOW and repeat:
As the sun shines so can I.
I release the need to be perfect.
I choose to switch on to the new and exciting experiences that life holds for me.

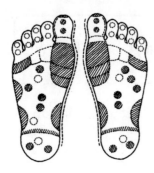

Zone Treatment

Each day, massage all your glands and organs; this will keep you super fit.

5

Other Applications

THE three-point system of Color Zone Therapy can be employed just as effectively in other areas of life; we have found that it works equally well for the treatment of children and the elderly, and for dealing with emotional issues that arise from relationships.

TREATING CHILDREN

Children respond extremely well to Color Zone Therapy, and they react to Zone Therapy treatment with elfin delight from the age of six months onwards. Remember that if you can keep every gland and organ functioning at 100 percent, then you can guarantee perfect health, and if your child is brought up on Zone Therapy techniques, the toxins, poisons, additives and colorings which destroy the body's defenses are being eliminated on a daily basis.

Children can also very quickly learn how to treat themselves and treat others, and it is a revelation to see them at work.

When you begin to give your child treatment, always start by rubbing the feet very gently, and learn how to treat the nerve endings kindly. This way, you build up a rapport, and the child will always look forward to the treatment. You will never regret introducing your child to Zone Therapy.

Children also respond extremely well to color; they are naturals. If you have a sick child at home, just present them with a box of paints or crayons, or colored pieces of material or card, and they will automatically choose the color that is right for their healing. In America, much research has been focused on the support of color in childcare; for instance, they have discovered that bathing a newborn baby in a blue light will effectively counteract the effects of jaundice. This approach has proved especially popular, because the required effect can be achieved without the use of drugs.

From birth until sixteen years age, children need pure red light—this is the color that is absorbed most by the system for speedy growth. But if a child has a temperature, a blue light in the bedroom will help bring it down. If the color purple is to be used for healing with the young, it should be used with extreme caution. The under-tens should not be exposed to it at all.

Color can be introduced easily to a child through diet, clothing and decor as well as by lighting. And you don't have to be an expert to harness the simple use of color. For instance, if your child is facing a difficult exam, you can help at this particular time with the use of the color yellow. Your child may well be sitting at a desk all day, and this will bring about sluggishness of the system, which can also result in constipation. In this case, use yellow food and decor, and yellow solarized water, to aid elimination and to stimulate the mind and the circulation. (To make yellow solarized water, wrap a piece of yellow cellophane around a glass of pure water. Put the glass on a window ledge, in the sunlight, and leave for four to six hours. Drink slowly. Do not drink *yellow* solarized water after 6:00pm).

Use the following three-step treatment with infants and children.

TREATMENT FOR INFANTS AND CHILDREN

Healing color (for both sexes, up to seven years) PINK
Healing color (over seven years, girls) PINK
Healing color (over seven years, boys) BLUE

Hold the child's foot, and gently massage it. Ask the child to think PINK, or else encourage him or her to color PINK on to a sheet of paper, or cuddle a PINK toy or blanket; alternatively, any PINK clothing can be worn. The child can also be encouraged to sing a favorite song or nursery rhyme. Continue to gently massage the foot all over, then repeat on the other foot.

TREATMENT FOR THE OLDER PERSON

As we move on in years, it can become a full-time job just to remain mobile and active, and prevent that slide down into inertia; we need a simple way of keeping in peak condition.

Just as the child of up to sixteen years needs the color red to further growth, so red is again the appropriate color here. It provides the key to keeping and maintaining health. Red is the life-force ray; as the years pass, it will help us to keep that zest, energy and drive, and the spark within us still firing.

Older people are also prone to hypothermia, so keep the red coming to guard against this too—our grandparents weren't fools for wearing their red flannel nightwear to keep them warm in winter!

Elimination can again become a problem in the later years, just as it can be for the studying teenager; it is vital to keep the system free of toxins by aiding elimination. Then again, the eyesight also fades; individual colors such as yellow for elimination and purple for the eyesight can both also be focused upon as general all-round healing colors.

Use the following three-step treatment to keep mobility of body and joy of spirit.

REJUVENATION

Healing color **ORANGE**

Underlying Negative Mental and Emotional Attitude
Eliminate:
I'm afraid of getting
OLD.
I'm afraid of being SICK
and unable to look after
MYSELF.

Permanent Positive Thinking Replacement
Repeat:
I am perfect in all situations.
Every age has infinite possibilities.
My AGE is perfect.
I ENJOY every moment.

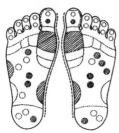

Zone Treatment

All men and women, from the age of fifty onwards, will gain great benefits from Color Zone Therapy; and because every organ and gland runs down with age, older people require the treatment on a daily basis.

Always start with the pituitary glands, then go on to the thyroid glands; give both of these a thorough going over. Then the adrenal and thymus glands need working on; the work you do on these is the most important. Then check out the liver, kidney, heart and spleen. Men should then work on the prostate gland. Women should work on the bladder.

If you work daily on these areas, it will transform your life and make you feel years younger.

EMOTIONAL RELATIONSHIPS

This three-step Color Zone Therapy treatment is for the grief, bereavement, shock or loss that anyone may experience, whether it be from the passing of a loved one, from divorce or from the ending of a relationship.

LOSS

Healing color **ORANGE**

Underlying Negative Mental and Emotional Attitude
Eliminate:
I'm afraid of being LONELY.

Permanent Positive Thinking Replacement
Repeat:
I can have an acceptance of that which
cannot be CHANGED.
I surrender to the law of the
DIVINE WILL.

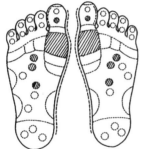

Zone Treatment
Work on the thyroid and parathyroid glands first. Then treat the pituitary gland centre, on the big toe. Also work on the nervous system, and the thymus and adrenal glands. Treatment should be given for five minutes on each foot, or until all discomfort disappears, twice a day.

In this book, we have introduced you to the first stages of finding the real you. If you practice Color Zone Therapy faithfully, it will open up an entire new world for you.

INDEX

For specific ailments see A-Z section, pages 57-162.

BOOKS BY THE CROSSING PRESS

The Alexander Technique and Beyond: *Moving Toward a More Balanced Expression of the Whole Self*
by Glen Park

The Alexander Technique has long been recognized throughout the world as a powerful method for unlearning unconscious, habitual behavior, alleviating physical and mental stress, and encouraging personal growth and transformation. In *The Alexander Technique and Beyond*, Glen Park makes it available to us in exciting new ways.
• $18.95• ISBN 089594-918-0

All Women Are Healers: *A Comprehensive Guide to Natural Healing*
By Diane Stein

A wealth of "how-to" information on various healing methods including Reiki, reflexology, polarity balancing, and homeopathy, intended to teach women to take control of their bodies and lives.
$14.95 • Paper • 0-89594-409-X

Chakras and Their Archetypes: *Uniting Energy Awareness and Spiritual Growth*
By Ambika Wauters

Linking classic archetypes to the seven chakras in the human energy system can reveal unconscious ways of behaving. Wauters helps us understand where our energy is blocked, which attitudes or emotional issues are responsible, and how to then transcend our limitations, make healthy choices, release creativity, and heal our pasts.
• $16.95 • ISBN 0-89594-891-5

Channeling for Everyone: *A Safe Step-by-Step Guide to Developing Your Intuition and Psychic Awareness*
by Tony Neate

Tony Neate's *Channeling for Everyone* is a clear, concise guide to developing that sensitivity. It provides us with a safe, step-by-step series of exercises to prepare for and begin to practice channeling.
• $12.95• ISBN 089594-922-9

Color and Crystals, A Journey Through the Chakras: *Healing with Color and Stones*
By Joy Gardner Gordon

Healing with stones, color, and tarot archetypes.
$12.95 • Paper • 0-89594-258-5

Essential Reiki: *A Complete Guide to an Ancient Healing Art*
By Diane Stein

While no book can replace the directly received Reiki attunements, *Essential Reiki* provides everything else that the healer, practitioner, and the teacher of this system needs, including full information on all three degrees of Reiki, most of it in print for the first time.
$18.95 • Paper • 0-89594-736-6

Handbook of Natural Therapies: *Exploring the Spiral of Healing*
by Marcia Starck

When we are troubled by an ailment not suited to treatment by allopathic or conventional Western medicine, what can we do? Whom do we turn to? Marcia Starck discusses nearly fifty therapies that can be used in a holistic approach to health.
• $14.95• ISBN 089594-869-9

The Healing Energy of Your Hands
By Michael Bradford

The techniques described are so simple that anyone, even a child, can begin to sense and work with healing energy.
$12.95 • Paper • 0-89594-781-1

Healing with Chinese Herbs
Lesley Tierra, L. Ac., Dip. Ac.

Expert practitioner Lesley Tierra shows how certain tonic herbs have been used by the Chinese for over 4,000 years to increase vitality and strengthen the body's natural functions. Tierra lists over 100 herbs, outlining their therapeutic uses and explaining how prescriptions are tailored to each patient's constitutional strength and particular condition.
$14.95 • Paper • 0-89594-829-X

BOOKS BY THE CROSSING PRESS

Healing with Gemstones and Crystals
By Diane Stein

Provides a complete guide to healing the body, mind, and spirit with the aid of gemstones and crystals. Practitioners as well as beginners will find a wealth of information and instructions on every page.
$14.95 • Paper • 0-89594-831-1

The Healing Voice: *Traditional & Contemporary Toning, Chanting and Singing*
By Joy Gardner Gordon

"In a fascinating blend of comparative anthropology, spiritual autobiography, and how-to, Gardner-Gordon asserts that most religious traditions have recognized the spiritual and biomedical efficacy of chanting and other forms of "toning" but acknowledges as well that Judeo-Christian culture slights this powerful means of contact between mind and body and between mind-body and the divine." —*Booklist*
$12.95 • Paper • 0-89594-571-1

The Sevenfold Journey: *Reclaiming Mind, Body & Spirit Through the Chakras*
By Anodea Judith and Selene Vega

Combining yoga, movement, psychotherapy, and ritual, the authors weave ancient and modern wisdom into a powerful tapestry of techniques for facilitating personal growth and healing.
• $18.95 • Paper ISBN 0-89594-574-6

Your Body Speaks Your Mind: *How Your Thoughts and Emotions Affect Your Health*
By Debbie Shapiro

Debbie Shapiro examines the intimate connection between the mind and body revealing insights into how our unresolved thoughts and feelings affect our health. This healing guide explores the structural body from the head to the toes, and the inner relationship of each part.
• $14.95 • ISBN 0-89594-893-1

To receive a current catalog from The Crossing Press
please call toll-free, 800-777-1048. (Prices subject to change.)
Visit our Web site on the Internet: www. crossingpress.com